LIVING FULLY

A Compassionate Guide to End-of-Life Choices, Caregiving, and Finding Meaning in Every Chapter of Life

Felicia Ward

LIVING FULLY

Copyright © 2025 by Felicia Ward.

All rights reserved. No part of this book may be reproduced, stored in a retrieval system, or transmitted in any form or by any means, electronic, mechanical, photocopying, recording, or otherwise, without prior written permission from the publisher, except for brief quotations embodied in critical reviews and certain other noncommercial uses permitted by copyright law.

LIVING FULLY

TABLE OF CONTENTS

Introduction..8
Chapter 1 - Redefining Independence: The Myths of Self-Sufficiency..12
Chapter 2 - When Stability Shifts: The Fragility of Control.......17
Chapter 3 - Facing the Unknown: The First Steps Toward Acceptance..22
Chapter 4 - The Weight of Choices: Balancing Freedom and Responsibility..27
Chapter 5 - The Role of Vulnerability in Strength.....................33
Chapter 6 - Seeking Help Without Shame................................38
Chapter 7 - The Power of a Listening Ear: Building Emotional Support Systems..44
Chapter 8: The Role of Professional Care: Doctors, Nurses, and the Hospice Team..50
Chapter 9 - Caregiving Essentials: Compassion Without Burnout..56
Chapter 10: Creating a Circle of Care: Family, Friends, and Community..62
Chapter 11: Coping with Terminal Diagnoses: A Path Forward.68
Chapter 12 - Grief as a Journey: From Denial to Acceptance....74
Chapter 13 - Emotional Healing: Finding Peace Amid Loss.......79
Chapter 14 - Confronting Fear: The Courage to Face Mortality...85
Chapter 15: Spiritual and Emotional Comfort: The Search for Inner Peace..90
Chapter 16: Palliative Care: Prioritizing Comfort and Quality of Life..95
Chapter 17: Hospice Care: A Compassionate Alternative to Prolonging Pain..101
Chapter 18: Difficult Conversations: Breaking the Silence Around Death..107

Chapter 19 - The Legacy We Leave Behind: Creating Meaning in Final Days...114

Chapter 20: Planning Ahead: Legal and Practical Considerations for End-of-Life.. 121

Chapter 21: Living Fully Until the End: Embracing Joy in Small Moments...127

Chapter 22 - The Gift of Letting Go: Finding Freedom in Acceptance.. 133

Chapter 23 - Guiding Loved Ones Through Grief and Bereavement..139

Chapter 24 - A Better Ending: Designing a Death That Aligns with Your Values.. 145

Chapter 25 - The Journey Beyond Loss: Hope and Renewal After Goodbye.. 151

LIVING FULLY

Introduction

Life is a journey of profound transitions—moments of joy, periods of struggle, and inevitable chapters of loss. It is a journey that demands courage, vulnerability, and the capacity to embrace the unknown. Yet, in a society that often avoids discussing mortality, we are rarely equipped to navigate the complexities of aging, caregiving, and end-of-life choices with clarity and compassion. This book, Living Fully: A Compassionate Guide to End-of-Life Choices, Caregiving, and Finding Meaning in Every Chapter of Life, is an invitation to explore these realities with openness, dignity, and hope.

As human beings, we are naturally inclined to seek control over our lives. We plan, we prepare, and we strive for independence, often equating self-sufficiency with strength. However, the reality of life is that control is fleeting, and independence is interwoven with interdependence. Whether through aging, illness, or the caregiving of a loved one, we all encounter moments that challenge our notions of self-reliance. These moments, though difficult, offer opportunities for growth, connection, and transformation.

This book is born from a desire to provide a roadmap for these transitions. It is a guide for those facing the uncertainty of a terminal diagnosis, for caregivers navigating the emotional and physical demands of supporting a loved one, and for anyone seeking to live fully in the face of life's impermanence. It is a resource for finding meaning in vulnerability, strength in community, and peace in the choices that shape our final chapters.

Living Fully is structured to address the multifaceted experiences of life's later stages, offering practical guidance, emotional support, and philosophical reflections. It begins by challenging cultural myths about independence and self-sufficiency, encouraging readers to redefine these concepts in ways that honor both autonomy and connection. As the book unfolds, it delves into the delicate balance between freedom and responsibility, the role of vulnerability in strength, and the transformative power of seeking help and building emotional support systems.

Caregiving, one of life's most demanding yet meaningful roles, is explored in depth. The book provides insights into navigating this journey with compassion while avoiding burnout, offering strategies for establishing boundaries, creating a circle of care, and fostering moments of connection. It acknowledges the emotional weight of caregiving and emphasizes the importance of self-care as a foundation for sustainable support.

For those facing terminal diagnoses or supporting loved ones through this experience, Living Fully offers a compassionate perspective on end-of-life planning, hospice care, and the search for meaning in final days. It encourages readers to engage in open conversations about death and dying, to articulate their values and wishes, and to embrace the legacy they wish to leave behind. By addressing these topics with honesty and sensitivity, the book seeks to demystify the end-of-life experience and empower readers to approach it with grace and intention.

At its heart, Living Fully is a celebration of human connection. It is a reminder that even in the face of loss and uncertainty, we are not alone. Our lives are enriched by the relationships we cultivate, the communities we build, and the love we share. This book invites readers to lean into these connections, to find strength in vulnerability, and to embrace the interdependence that defines the human experience.

Throughout these pages, you will encounter stories of resilience, practical advice, and reflections on the beauty and fragility of life. These narratives are not meant to prescribe a singular path but to inspire readers to chart their own course, guided by their values, relationships, and aspirations. Whether you are a caregiver, a patient, or someone seeking to understand life's transitions more deeply, this book offers tools and insights to help you navigate the journey with compassion and clarity.

The title of this book, Living Fully, is both an aspiration and a call to action. It is an invitation to embrace life in all its complexity—to find joy in small moments, to seek meaning in challenges, and to approach the end of life not with fear, but with a sense of purpose and peace. Living fully means acknowledging our mortality while celebrating the relationships, experiences, and choices that make life meaningful.

As you embark on this journey through the pages of this book, I encourage you to approach it with an open heart and mind. Allow yourself to reflect on your own experiences, fears, and hopes. Engage with the stories and insights shared here, and consider how they might inform your own path. Most importantly, remember that living fully is not about perfection or control; it is about embracing the beauty of life's impermanence and finding meaning in every chapter.

Let us walk this path together, with compassion, courage, and a commitment to living fully until the very end.

Chapter 1 - Redefining Independence: The Myths of Self-Sufficiency

Independence is a cherished ideal in our culture, often equated with strength, success, and personal achievement. We celebrate the lone wolf who conquers challenges through sheer willpower, the self-made individual who navigates the world without assistance, and the stoic figure who faces adversity head-on, unyielding and unbroken. Yet, as we journey through life, we inevitably encounter moments that challenge this notion of self-sufficiency, particularly as we age or face illness. The myths surrounding independence can obscure a deeper truth: that true strength often lies in our ability to acknowledge our vulnerabilities and seek support from others. In this exploration, we will unravel the complexities of independence, examining how our understanding of self-sufficiency can evolve in the face of life's inevitable transitions.

Consider the elderly man who has spent decades living alone in his modest home, fiercely proud of his ability to manage on his own. He rises each morning, brews his coffee, and tends to his garden, the fruits of his labor a testament to his independence. Yet, when a sudden illness leaves him weak and disoriented, the very foundation of his self-sufficiency begins to crumble. The simple tasks that once defined his daily routine—grocery shopping, maintaining the yard, or even preparing a meal—become Herculean challenges. It is in these moments of fragility that the myths of independence are laid bare, revealing the complexities of human existence. The man may grapple with feelings of failure or shame, believing that needing help diminishes his worth. However, this perspective overlooks the reality that interdependence is a fundamental aspect of the human experience, one that can lead to deeper connections and a more profound sense of belonging.

The tension between self-sufficiency and dependence is particularly palpable in caregiving scenarios. Caregivers often navigate a delicate balance, striving to provide support while respecting the autonomy of their loved ones. The elderly woman, for instance, may resist assistance with bathing or dressing, clinging to her sense of agency even as her physical capabilities wane. In these moments, caregivers face the challenge of honoring their loved ones' desires while recognizing the practical realities of their situation. The struggle is not merely about tasks or responsibilities; it is a profound negotiation of identity, dignity, and love. The caregiver must approach these conversations with empathy and patience, understanding that the desire for independence is deeply rooted in our humanity. It is essential to frame assistance not as a loss of autonomy but as a collaborative effort—a partnership that honors both the caregiver's and the care recipient's needs.

Moreover, the societal narrative surrounding independence often neglects the importance of community and connection. We live in a world that increasingly emphasizes individualism, where self-reliance is celebrated at the expense of communal ties. Yet, research consistently shows that social support is a critical determinant of well-being, particularly in times of crisis. The elderly man who once relished his solitude may find solace in the company of neighbors or friends who offer to help with errands or simply share a cup of coffee. In these interactions, he discovers that vulnerability can foster intimacy, and that asking for help can lead to unexpected joys. The myths of independence begin to dissolve, replaced by a richer understanding of what it means to live fully in community with others.

As we navigate the complexities of life, we must also confront the realities of our mortality. The prospect of illness or death can provoke existential questions about what it means to live a meaningful life. For many, the fear of losing independence is intertwined with the fear of losing identity. When faced with a terminal diagnosis, individuals may grapple with the loss of control over their bodies and lives, leading to feelings of helplessness. Yet, it is precisely in these moments of uncertainty that we have the opportunity to redefine what independence means. Rather than viewing it solely through the lens of self-sufficiency, we can embrace a broader understanding that encompasses emotional resilience, the courage to face vulnerability, and the willingness to accept help from others.

In this context, the role of healthcare professionals becomes paramount. Doctors, nurses, and hospice workers serve not only as providers of medical care but as facilitators of meaningful conversations about independence and interdependence. They can help patients articulate their values and preferences, guiding them in making choices that align with their desires for dignity and autonomy. The physician who listens attentively to a patient's concerns about losing independence can validate those feelings while also providing reassurance that support is available. This collaborative approach fosters a sense of agency, allowing individuals to reclaim their narratives even in the face of daunting challenges.

Ultimately, redefining independence requires a shift in mindset—a recognition that our lives are not solely defined by our ability to stand alone, but by our capacity to connect with others. It invites us to embrace the paradox that vulnerability can coexist with strength, and that asking for help is not a sign of weakness but a testament to our humanity. In navigating the complexities of life, loss, and the journey to peace, we must challenge the myths of self-sufficiency and celebrate the beauty of interdependence. By doing so, we open ourselves to deeper relationships, richer experiences, and a more profound understanding of what it means to live fully in every chapter of our lives. As we embark on this journey together, let us remember that true independence is not about isolation, but about the courage to reach out, to lean on one another, and to find strength in our shared humanity.

Chapter 2 - When Stability Shifts: The Fragility of Control

Life is a delicate tapestry, woven together with threads of stability and the unpredictable nature of existence. We often take for granted the routines that provide us with a sense of control—morning rituals, work schedules, family dinners. These elements of our lives create a comforting illusion of permanence, a semblance of mastery over our circumstances. Yet, as we navigate the complexities of aging, illness, and impending loss, we begin to realize just how fragile this sense of control truly is. The moment we confront the reality of a loved one's declining health or our own mortality, the ground beneath us shifts, and we are left grappling with the disorienting truth that stability is often just a fleeting state.

Consider the elderly man who has lived independently for decades, managing his own affairs, tending to his garden, and enjoying the simple pleasures of life. One day, he trips and falls, fracturing his hip. In an instant, the stability he relied upon crumbles, and he finds himself in a hospital bed, surrounded by unfamiliar faces and sterile white walls. The autonomy he once enjoyed is replaced by a dependency on nurses, doctors, and family members who must now make decisions on his behalf. This shift can be jarring, not just for him but for everyone involved. The very essence of who he is feels threatened as he navigates this new landscape of fragility. He may resist assistance, clinging to the remnants of his independence, but the reality is that control has slipped through his fingers, leaving him to confront the vulnerabilities he had long denied.

In these moments of upheaval, the questions that arise are profound and unsettling. What does it mean to lose control over one's life? How do we reconcile the desire for independence with the reality of needing help? These inquiries are not merely theoretical; they penetrate the core of our existence and challenge our perceptions of self-worth and identity. For many, the act of asking for help feels like a surrender, an admission of defeat. Yet, in truth, it is a courageous step toward acceptance—a recognition that we are all interconnected and that our lives are not solely our own to manage. The intricate web of relationships we cultivate throughout our lives is designed to support us in times of need, yet the societal narrative often encourages a stoic self-sufficiency that can be isolating and detrimental.

As we navigate the shifting sands of control, it is essential to acknowledge the emotional weight that accompanies these changes. The elderly man in the hospital may feel a profound sense of loss—not just of his physical capabilities but also of his identity. He may grapple with feelings of inadequacy, perceiving himself as a burden to his loved ones. These emotions are common, yet they are often compounded by the fear of becoming irrelevant or forgotten. In our culture, where independence is celebrated, the loss of that independence can evoke feelings of shame and despair. It is crucial to create space for these emotions, allowing ourselves and our loved ones to express the grief associated with this loss. By doing so, we can foster an environment that encourages open dialogue about vulnerability, reinforcing the idea that needing help is a natural part of the human experience.

As we confront the fragility of control, we must also consider the role of caregivers in this narrative. Caregiving often emerges as a response to the shifting dynamics of independence, yet it can be a heavy burden to bear. Family members may find themselves thrust into the role of caregiver without warning, navigating the complexities of medical decisions, emotional support, and the logistics of daily care. This sudden shift can lead to feelings of overwhelm and inadequacy, as caregivers grapple with their own fears and uncertainties. The fragility of control extends beyond the individual facing health challenges; it envelops the entire family unit, altering relationships and reshaping dynamics. Open communication becomes paramount in these situations, allowing caregivers to express their struggles and seek support from others. Just as the elderly man must learn to accept help, caregivers must also recognize the importance of their own well-being. They must understand that they cannot pour from an empty cup and that seeking assistance is not a sign of weakness but rather an acknowledgment of their shared humanity.

As we delve deeper into the complexities of control and vulnerability, we must also confront the societal structures that shape our understanding of aging and illness. Our culture often glorifies youth and independence while stigmatizing the natural process of aging and the need for assistance. This narrative creates a chasm between those who are aging and those who are not, fostering an environment of isolation and fear. To bridge this gap, we must cultivate a culture of compassion that embraces the realities of life's fragility. This involves challenging societal norms and redefining what it means to live fully, regardless of age or ability. By fostering a more inclusive community that values interdependence, we can create a supportive framework that honors the dignity of all individuals, regardless of their circumstances.

In moments of profound uncertainty, we often find ourselves searching for meaning. The fragility of control can lead us to reconsider our priorities and values, prompting us to seek deeper connections with ourselves and others. As we navigate the complexities of life, loss, and the journey to peace, we must remember that the essence of living fully lies not in the pursuit of control but in the acceptance of life's inherent unpredictability. Embracing vulnerability allows us to forge authentic connections, to share our fears and hopes, and to support one another in moments of need. It is through these connections that we can find solace and strength, reminding ourselves that we are not alone in our struggles.

Ultimately, the fragility of control teaches us profound lessons about the nature of existence. Life is a series of ebbs and flows, a dance between independence and interdependence. As we navigate the shifting tides, we must learn to embrace the beauty of vulnerability and the strength that comes from asking for help. In doing so, we create a more compassionate world—one that recognizes the value of every individual, regardless of their circumstances. The journey toward acceptance may be fraught with challenges, but it is also rich with opportunities for growth, connection, and ultimately, peace. As we face the unknown, let us do so with open hearts, ready to embrace the complexities of life, loss, and the shared human experience.

Chapter 3 - Facing the Unknown: The First Steps Toward Acceptance

In the quiet moments that follow a diagnosis or the onset of a serious illness, the world seems to shift beneath our feet. It is a disorienting experience, akin to standing on the edge of a precipice, peering into an abyss that is both terrifying and profoundly unknown. The fear of what lies ahead can be paralyzing, but it is in these moments that we must begin the difficult journey towards acceptance. Acceptance does not mean resignation; rather, it is the process of coming to terms with our reality, of acknowledging the uncertainty that life presents, and of finding a way to navigate through it. This chapter explores the initial steps toward embracing the unknown, a journey that requires courage, vulnerability, and a willingness to confront our deepest fears.

When faced with the prospect of loss—whether it be the loss of health, independence, or life itself—the instinctual response is often to retreat into denial. Denial serves as a protective mechanism, shielding us from the emotional weight of our circumstances. We may find ourselves uttering phrases like "This can't be happening to me" or "I'm sure it will get better." While these thoughts may provide temporary solace, they ultimately delay the inevitable confrontation with reality. The first step toward acceptance is to acknowledge the truth of our situation, however uncomfortable it may be. This acknowledgment does not have to be a grand declaration; it can be as simple as allowing ourselves to feel the full spectrum of our emotions—fear, anger, sadness, and even moments of clarity and peace.

Acceptance is often mistaken for passivity, but it is, in fact, an active process. It requires us to engage with our circumstances, to ask difficult questions, and to seek understanding. What does this diagnosis mean for my life? How will it change my daily routines, my relationships, and my sense of self? These questions can be daunting, yet they are essential for moving forward. As we grapple with the reality of our situation, we may also find ourselves reflecting on the values that have shaped our lives. What truly matters to us? What brings us joy? What do we wish to prioritize in the time we have left? These reflections can serve as a guiding light, illuminating a path through the darkness of uncertainty.

In this process, it is crucial to recognize that we are not alone. The human experience is inherently interconnected, and the journey toward acceptance is one that is often shared. Engaging with family, friends, and support networks can provide a sense of community and belonging. Conversations about our fears and hopes can foster deeper connections, allowing us to feel less isolated in our struggles. It is in these exchanges that we may find unexpected sources of strength and resilience. We learn that vulnerability is not a weakness but rather a profound act of courage that can lead to healing and understanding.

As we begin to accept the unknown, we may also find ourselves confronting the narratives we have constructed around death and dying. Society often portrays these experiences in stark and clinical terms, emphasizing loss and grief without acknowledging the richness of life that persists even in the face of mortality. It is essential to challenge these narratives and to seek out stories that resonate with our own experiences. Reading memoirs, listening to podcasts, and engaging with others who have navigated similar paths can provide valuable insights. These stories remind us that while the unknown can be frightening, it can also be a space for growth, reflection, and transformation.

The journey toward acceptance is not linear; it is filled with ups and downs, moments of clarity interspersed with doubt. There will be days when we feel empowered and at peace with our choices, and there will be days when the weight of uncertainty feels unbearable. It is important to allow ourselves the grace to experience this ebb and flow without judgment. Embracing the unknown means giving ourselves permission to feel whatever arises, to honor our emotional landscape, and to seek support when needed. It is a reminder that we are human, that we are allowed to experience the full range of emotions that come with facing our mortality.

In the midst of this journey, we may also discover the power of mindfulness and presence. Practicing mindfulness allows us to anchor ourselves in the present moment, to appreciate the beauty of life as it unfolds, even amid uncertainty. Simple practices such as deep breathing, meditation, or spending time in nature can help us cultivate a sense of calm and clarity. These moments of stillness can serve as a refuge from the chaos of our thoughts, reminding us that life continues to hold meaning and beauty, even in its most challenging chapters.

As we navigate the unknown, it is essential to cultivate a sense of agency. Even when faced with circumstances beyond our control, we can make choices that align with our values and priorities. This might involve having difficult conversations with loved ones about our wishes for end-of-life care, seeking out palliative services that prioritize comfort, or simply choosing to engage in activities that bring us joy. Each choice we make, no matter how small, can empower us to reclaim a sense of control over our lives, reinforcing the idea that we are not merely passive recipients of our circumstances but active participants in our journey.

The process of acceptance is also intertwined with the concept of legacy. As we confront the unknown, we may find ourselves reflecting on the mark we wish to leave on the world. What do we want our loved ones to remember about us? What values do we hope to impart? Engaging with these questions can inspire us to live more fully in the present, to express our love and gratitude, and to create meaningful experiences with those we cherish. It is through this lens of legacy that we can find purpose in our journey, even as we face the inevitability of loss.

Ultimately, the journey toward acceptance is about embracing the complexity of life itself. It is about acknowledging that while we cannot control every aspect of our existence, we can choose how we respond to the challenges we face. It is about finding strength in vulnerability, seeking connection in our struggles, and discovering meaning in the midst of uncertainty. As we take these initial steps toward acceptance, we may find that the unknown is not solely a source of fear but also a canvas upon which we can paint our most authentic selves. In the face of life's fragility, we have the opportunity to live fully, to love deeply, and to navigate our journey with grace and courage.

Chapter 4 - The Weight of Choices: Balancing Freedom and Responsibility

As we navigate the complex terrain of life, the choices we face can feel both liberating and burdensome. The notion of freedom often carries with it an inherent weight—a weight that can become particularly pronounced in the context of end-of-life decisions. We are presented with a myriad of options, and while this abundance can feel empowering, it can also lead to a paralyzing sense of responsibility. The choices we make not only reflect our values and beliefs but also have profound implications for our loved ones, caregivers, and even the healthcare system. The challenge lies in balancing this freedom with the responsibility that comes with it, particularly as we confront the realities of mortality.

In our society, independence is often celebrated as a virtue. We are taught from a young age to strive for self-sufficiency, to make our own decisions, and to carve our own paths. However, as we age or face health challenges, the very concept of independence can become fraught with ambiguity. The desire to maintain control over one's life can clash with the need for assistance, leading to an internal struggle that can feel isolating. This tension is magnified when it comes to end-of-life choices, where the stakes are high, and the implications of our decisions are profound. We may find ourselves grappling with questions about how much autonomy we truly possess and how much we are willing to relinquish in the face of illness or impending death.

The weight of choices becomes particularly evident when we consider the various paths available for end-of-life care. Patients and families are often faced with decisions about treatment options, palliative care, hospice services, and even the choice to forgo aggressive interventions. Each option carries its own set of implications, not only for the patient but also for family members who may have differing opinions about what constitutes the "right" choice. The pressure to make the best decision can feel overwhelming, especially when the consequences of those choices are so significant. In these moments, the desire for autonomy can clash with the fear of making a wrong decision, leading to a state of paralysis where individuals may feel they are not only responsible for their own fate but also for the emotional well-being of those around them.

Moreover, the societal narrative around choice often emphasizes the importance of individual preferences, yet this narrative can overlook the interconnectedness of our lives. The choices we make do not exist in a vacuum; they ripple outward, affecting our families, friends, and caregivers. The burden of these choices can weigh heavily on both patients and their loved ones, creating a complex web of emotions that includes guilt, anxiety, and fear. It is essential to recognize that while we strive for independence, we are also part of a larger community, and our choices can either strengthen or strain those relationships. This realization can be both liberating and daunting, as it invites us to consider not only our own desires but also the needs and feelings of those around us.

As we grapple with these choices, it is crucial to cultivate an environment that encourages open dialogue about our values and preferences. This can be particularly challenging in a culture that often shies away from conversations about death and dying. However, fostering these discussions can help alleviate some of the weight of decision-making, allowing individuals to express their wishes and concerns while also considering the perspectives of their loved ones. By creating a safe space for these conversations, we can begin to navigate the complexities of choice with greater clarity and compassion. This process involves not only articulating our own desires but also actively listening to the hopes and fears of those who will be affected by our decisions.

In addition to fostering open communication, it is essential to seek out reliable sources of information and support when faced with difficult choices. The landscape of healthcare is often overwhelming, filled with medical jargon and complex treatment options that can leave patients and families feeling lost. Engaging with healthcare professionals who are skilled in end-of-life care can provide invaluable guidance, helping individuals to understand their options and the potential consequences of each choice. This collaboration can empower patients to make informed decisions that align with their values while alleviating some of the burdens of responsibility. It is important to remember that seeking help is not a sign of weakness; rather, it is an acknowledgment of the complexity of the situation we face.

As we navigate the weight of choices, it is also vital to recognize the role of hope in this process. Hope can be a powerful motivator, encouraging individuals to envision a future that aligns with their values and desires. However, hope can also be fraught with tension, particularly when it comes to end-of-life decisions. The desire for a miracle cure or a reversal of circumstances can sometimes cloud our judgment, leading us to make choices that may not be in our best interest. It is essential to balance hope with realism, acknowledging the limitations of our circumstances while also remaining open to the possibility of meaningful experiences in the time we have left. This delicate dance between hope and acceptance can help us navigate the weight of choices with greater ease, allowing us to find peace amid uncertainty.

Ultimately, the journey through the weight of choices is deeply personal and often tumultuous. Each individual's experience is shaped by their values, beliefs, and relationships, making it essential to approach these decisions with compassion and understanding. While the burden of responsibility can feel heavy, it is important to remember that we are not alone in this journey. Our choices are intertwined with the lives of those we love, and by embracing the interconnectedness of our experiences, we can create a more supportive and compassionate environment for ourselves and those around us.

In conclusion, the weight of choices in the context of end-of-life decisions is a complex interplay of freedom and responsibility. As we navigate this terrain, we must strive to maintain open communication, seek reliable support, and balance hope with realism. By doing so, we can approach these choices with greater clarity and compassion, ultimately finding a path that honors our values while also considering the needs of our loved ones. It is through this delicate balance that we can begin to navigate the challenges of life, loss, and the journey to peace, embracing the richness of our experiences even in the face of uncertainty. The choices we make may shape our final chapters, but they also hold the potential to create meaning and connection in the lives of those we leave behind.

Chapter 5 - The Role of Vulnerability in Strength

Vulnerability is often perceived as a weakness, a chink in the armor of self-sufficiency that we so fervently strive to maintain. In a society that glorifies independence and self-reliance, admitting to our vulnerabilities can feel like a betrayal of our very identity. Yet, as we navigate the profound realities of life, loss, and the journey toward peace, it becomes increasingly clear that vulnerability is not a flaw to be hidden but rather a powerful source of strength. It is a bridge that connects us to one another, a reminder that we are not alone in our struggles. When we allow ourselves to be vulnerable, we create space for genuine connection, compassion, and understanding—elements that are essential in the face of life's most challenging moments.

Consider the experience of caregiving, often a role thrust upon us unexpectedly. The initial instinct might be to project confidence, to present ourselves as the unwavering pillar of support for our loved ones. Yet, the truth is that caregiving can be overwhelming, filled with uncertainty and emotional turmoil. In these moments, embracing our vulnerability can lead to deeper connections with those we are caring for. When we share our fears, our doubts, and our struggles, we invite others to do the same. This mutual openness fosters a sense of solidarity, transforming the caregiving experience into a shared journey rather than a solitary burden. The act of acknowledging our vulnerabilities allows us to build bridges of empathy, creating an environment where both caregivers and those receiving care can express their needs and emotions without fear of judgment.

The journey through illness, particularly terminal illness, is fraught with vulnerability for both patients and caregivers. Patients may grapple with the fear of losing their autonomy, the pain of their diagnosis, and the uncertainty of what lies ahead. Caregivers, on the other hand, may wrestle with feelings of helplessness, anxiety about their loved one's suffering, and the weight of impending loss. In such circumstances, vulnerability can serve as a catalyst for meaningful conversations. When patients and caregivers share their fears and hopes, they often find clarity in their shared experiences. This dialogue can illuminate the path forward, allowing both parties to express their wishes for care and comfort in a way that honors their individual needs and desires. It is through vulnerability that the often-taboo subjects of death and dying can be approached with honesty and compassion, paving the way for more profound and fulfilling relationships during life's final chapters.

Moreover, embracing vulnerability can enhance our ability to find meaning even in the most painful experiences. When we confront our fears and uncertainties, we open ourselves to the possibility of growth and transformation. The act of being vulnerable encourages us to reflect on what truly matters—our relationships, our values, and the legacy we wish to leave behind. In the face of loss, this introspection can lead to a deeper understanding of ourselves and our place in the world. It can inspire us to engage more fully with life, to cherish the small moments of joy that can coexist with grief. By acknowledging our vulnerabilities, we allow ourselves to be present, to experience the fullness of our emotions, and to find beauty even amid sorrow.

As we navigate our own vulnerabilities, it is also essential to recognize and honor the vulnerabilities of those we care for. Each individual's experience with illness and loss is unique, shaped by their personal history, relationships, and coping mechanisms. By approaching others with empathy and an open heart, we create an environment where they feel safe to express their fears and desires. This practice not only strengthens our relationships but also empowers those we care for to take an active role in their own care. When patients feel heard and understood, they are more likely to articulate their needs and preferences, leading to a more patient-centered approach to care that respects their dignity and autonomy.

In the context of end-of-life care, vulnerability plays a crucial role in facilitating difficult conversations about death and dying. Many individuals fear discussing their wishes for end-of-life care, often due to societal taboos surrounding death. However, when we embrace our own vulnerabilities, we can create a safe space for these conversations to take place. Sharing our thoughts about our mortality can inspire others to do the same, allowing for a more comprehensive understanding of what it means to live fully until the end. These discussions can encompass everything from preferences for medical interventions to desires for how we wish to be remembered. In doing so, we empower ourselves and our loved ones to make informed choices that align with our values and beliefs, ultimately leading to a more peaceful and meaningful end-of-life experience.

It is also important to recognize that vulnerability is not a destination but a continuous journey. Life is inherently unpredictable, and our circumstances can change in an instant. As we navigate the complexities of caregiving and end-of-life decisions, we must remain open to the ebb and flow of our emotions. There will be days when we feel strong and capable, and others when we are overwhelmed with doubt and fear. In these moments, it is essential to practice self-compassion, to remind ourselves that vulnerability is a natural part of the human experience. By acknowledging our feelings without judgment, we create space for healing and growth. This self-awareness can also inform our interactions with others, allowing us to approach their vulnerabilities with greater empathy and understanding.

In conclusion, the role of vulnerability in strength is a profound and transformative concept that can significantly impact our experiences with life, loss, and caregiving. By embracing our vulnerabilities, we foster deeper connections, enhance our understanding of ourselves and others, and create an environment where meaningful conversations can flourish. In a world that often prioritizes self-sufficiency, it is essential to recognize that true strength lies in our ability to be open, honest, and compassionate—both with ourselves and with those we care for. As we navigate the complexities of end-of-life choices and the emotional landscape of grief, may we find solace in the knowledge that vulnerability is not a weakness to be feared but a powerful force that can guide us toward greater peace and fulfillment in every chapter of life.

Chapter 6 - Seeking Help Without Shame

In a society that often equates independence with strength, the act of seeking help can feel like an admission of failure. We are taught to be self-sufficient, to pull ourselves up by our bootstraps, to face challenges head-on without burdening others. This cultural narrative is particularly pronounced when it comes to caregiving and end-of-life decisions, where the stakes are high, and emotions run deep. Yet, as we navigate the complexities of life, loss, and the journey to peace, we must confront the uncomfortable truth: asking for help is not a sign of weakness; it is an essential part of the human experience. Embracing this notion can be transformative, allowing us to foster connections that enrich our lives and the lives of those we care for.

The reluctance to seek help often stems from a fear of vulnerability. We worry that by revealing our struggles, we will be perceived as inadequate or less capable. This fear is compounded by the societal pressure to maintain a façade of control and composure, especially when faced with the profound challenges of illness or caregiving. However, vulnerability is not the enemy; it is the doorway to deeper relationships and authentic support. When we allow ourselves to be seen—flaws and all—we invite others to step into our lives, offering their compassion and understanding. In the context of caregiving, this can mean reaching out to friends, family, or support groups to share our burdens and seek guidance. It can also involve seeking professional help, whether through counseling, therapy, or hospice services. In doing so, we not only lighten our load but also create a space for others to share their own struggles, fostering a culture of mutual support.

One of the most profound lessons I have learned in my journey through caregiving and loss is that asking for help can lead to unexpected gifts. When my father was diagnosed with terminal cancer, I was overwhelmed by the weight of his illness and the responsibility of caring for him. I initially believed that I could manage everything on my own, that I should be strong and stoic for his sake. But as the days stretched into weeks, and the demands of caregiving intensified, I found myself increasingly isolated and exhausted. It was during this time that I finally broke down and reached out to a close friend, sharing my fears and frustrations. To my surprise, my friend responded not with pity, but with empathy and understanding. She offered to sit with my father while I took a much-needed break, and in that moment, I realized that asking for help was not an act of surrender but a pathway to resilience.

The act of seeking help can take many forms, and it is important to recognize that it does not always require grand gestures or formal arrangements. Sometimes, it is the small acts of kindness from friends and family that make the most significant difference. A simple phone call, a home-cooked meal, or a listening ear can provide a lifeline during the most challenging times. These gestures remind us that we are not alone in our struggles and that there is a community of support ready to rally around us. In the context of caregiving, it can be particularly helpful to create a network of support that includes not only family and friends but also professionals who can provide guidance and assistance. This might include doctors, nurses, social workers, or hospice teams who specialize in end-of-life care. By embracing a holistic approach to support, we can cultivate a comprehensive safety net that addresses both our physical and emotional needs.

It is also essential to challenge the stigma surrounding the need for help. In many cultures, there is an ingrained belief that seeking assistance is a sign of failure or inadequacy. This stigma can be especially pronounced in the context of caregiving, where the expectation is often to be selfless and unwavering. However, acknowledging our limitations is not a weakness; it is an act of courage. By reframing the narrative around help-seeking, we can empower ourselves and others to embrace vulnerability as a strength. It is through this lens that we can begin to dismantle the barriers that prevent us from reaching out, creating a more compassionate and understanding environment for all.

As we navigate the complexities of life and loss, it is crucial to remember that seeking help is not a solitary journey. It is a collective experience that involves building connections and fostering relationships. Engaging with others who have faced similar challenges can provide invaluable insights and support. Support groups, whether in-person or online, offer a space for individuals to share their experiences and learn from one another. These gatherings can be a source of comfort, validation, and encouragement, reminding us that we are not alone in our struggles. In sharing our stories, we not only find solace but also contribute to a larger narrative of resilience and hope.

Moreover, seeking help does not mean relinquishing control or agency. Instead, it can enhance our ability to make informed decisions and advocate for ourselves and our loved ones. When we engage with professionals in the field of end-of-life care, we gain access to a wealth of knowledge and resources that can guide us through the complexities of the healthcare system. This collaboration can empower us to make choices that align with our values and preferences, ensuring that our voices are heard and respected. In this way, asking for help becomes an act of self-advocacy, reinforcing our commitment to living fully, even in the face of adversity.

The journey of caregiving and facing the end of life is fraught with uncertainty and emotional turmoil. It is natural to feel overwhelmed, anxious, or even resentful at times. However, by embracing the practice of seeking help, we can transform these feelings into opportunities for growth and connection. Each time we reach out, we create a ripple effect that can inspire others to do the same. In this way, we contribute to a culture of openness and support that transcends individual experiences, fostering a sense of community and belonging.

As we reflect on the importance of seeking help without shame, it is essential to recognize that this journey is deeply personal. Each individual will have their own unique path, shaped by their experiences, beliefs, and circumstances. What is most important is that we honor our own needs and the needs of those we care for. This may involve setting boundaries, prioritizing self-care, and recognizing when it is time to ask for assistance. By doing so, we can cultivate an environment that nurtures both our own well-being and that of our loved ones.

Ultimately, the act of seeking help is a testament to our humanity. It is a recognition that we are not meant to navigate life's challenges alone. In reaching out, we acknowledge our interconnectedness and the profound impact that relationships have on our lives. As we journey through the complexities of caregiving, loss, and acceptance, let us embrace the power of vulnerability and the strength that comes from asking for help. In doing so, we can create a legacy of compassion and understanding that will resonate far beyond our individual experiences, enriching the lives of those around us and fostering a deeper sense of connection in a world that often feels fragmented.

Chapter 7 - The Power of a Listening Ear: Building Emotional Support Systems

As we navigate the complex terrain of life, loss, and the journey to peace, we often overlook one of the most profound tools we have at our disposal: the power of a listening ear. In a world that often values productivity and self-sufficiency, we can mistakenly equate asking for help with weakness, or seek solace in the belief that we must carry our burdens alone. Yet, in times of grief, uncertainty, and transition, the act of sharing our thoughts, fears, and stories can be a lifeline, a means of connection that not only alleviates our emotional pain but also fosters a sense of community and understanding. The simple gift of listening can transform our experiences, turning isolation into connection, despair into hope.

Consider the moments when you have felt overwhelmed by sadness or uncertainty. Perhaps it was the day you received a terminal diagnosis, or the moment you realized that a loved one was slipping away. In those instances, the impulse to retreat into silence can be powerful. We often believe that our struggles are burdensome to others, that our grief is too heavy for anyone else to bear. However, the truth is that sharing our experiences can create opportunities for empathy and support that we might not have anticipated. When we open up, we invite others into our world, allowing them to share in our journey, and in turn, we give them the chance to express their own feelings of loss and fear. This exchange can be healing, both for the speaker and the listener.

The power of a listening ear is not just about the act of speaking; it is equally about the act of listening. In our fast-paced society, genuine listening has become a rare commodity. We often find ourselves distracted, our minds racing ahead to formulate responses rather than fully engaging with what the other person is saying. True listening requires presence, a willingness to set aside our own agendas and immerse ourselves in the emotions and experiences of another. It is about creating a safe space where vulnerability can flourish. When we listen with intention, we communicate to others that their feelings matter, that their stories are worthy of being heard. This validation can be profoundly comforting, especially in times of distress.

Building emotional support systems is not merely about finding someone to talk to; it is about cultivating relationships that foster mutual understanding and compassion. This can take many forms—friends, family members, support groups, or even professional therapists. Each of these connections offers a unique perspective, a different facet of understanding that can enrich our experience. For instance, a friend may provide a sense of camaraderie and shared experience, while a therapist can offer tools and strategies for coping with grief. Support groups, too, create a community of individuals who are walking similar paths, allowing for shared stories and collective healing. The key is to seek out those relationships that resonate with us, that make us feel seen and heard.

In the context of caregiving, the importance of emotional support systems becomes even more pronounced. Caregivers often find themselves in the role of both provider and protector, navigating the delicate balance of tending to the needs of their loved ones while grappling with their own emotions. The weight of responsibility can feel insurmountable, leading to feelings of isolation and burnout. Here, the act of reaching out becomes essential. Caregivers must not only recognize their own needs for support but also be willing to accept help from others. This might mean allowing family members to step in, seeking respite care, or simply confiding in a friend about the challenges they face. By doing so, caregivers can replenish their emotional reserves, enabling them to provide more compassionate care.

Moreover, the act of listening can also serve as a powerful tool for self-reflection. When we articulate our thoughts and feelings, we often gain clarity about our own experiences. Journaling, for example, can be a form of self-listening, allowing us to explore our emotions in a safe and private space. Conversations with trusted friends or family members can also facilitate this process, as they provide an opportunity to vocalize our fears and hopes, helping us to better understand our own needs. In this way, listening becomes a two-way street, a dynamic exchange that fosters growth and healing.

The importance of emotional support systems extends beyond the individual. As we cultivate our own networks of support, we also contribute to a culture that values connection and empathy. By sharing our experiences and encouraging others to do the same, we help to dismantle the stigma surrounding grief and vulnerability. We remind each other that it is okay to feel lost, to seek help, and to lean on one another during difficult times. This collective effort can create a ripple effect, inspiring others to build their own support systems and fostering a sense of community that can be a source of strength for all.

In the realm of end-of-life care, the power of a listening ear takes on an even deeper significance. Patients facing terminal diagnoses often grapple with profound existential questions, fears of the unknown, and the weight of unfinished business. In these moments, the act of listening can provide solace, a means of acknowledging their experiences without judgment. It is a chance for them to share their hopes, regrets, and dreams, to articulate what matters most in their final days. Caregivers and loved ones can play a crucial role in this process, offering their presence and attention as a form of support. By creating space for these conversations, we honor the dignity of those we care for, allowing them to express their fears and desires as they navigate the uncharted waters of mortality.

In this context, we must also recognize the importance of professional support systems, such as hospice and palliative care teams. These professionals are trained not only to manage physical symptoms but also to provide emotional and psychological support to patients and their families. They understand the complexities of grief and loss, and they can help facilitate conversations that might otherwise feel too daunting. By working alongside these professionals, we can enhance our own emotional support systems, ensuring that we have the tools and resources necessary to navigate the challenges of end-of-life care.

Ultimately, the power of a listening ear is a reminder that we are not alone in our struggles. It is an invitation to share our stories, to connect with others, and to seek comfort in the knowledge that our experiences are valid and worthy of being heard. In a world that often prioritizes independence and self-reliance, we must embrace the idea that vulnerability and connection are not signs of weakness but rather sources of strength. By building emotional support systems, we create a tapestry of relationships that enrich our lives, provide solace in times of grief, and foster a sense of belonging that transcends the challenges we face.

As we continue on our journey through life, loss, and the pursuit of peace, let us remember the transformative power of listening. Let us be willing to share our stories and to open ourselves to the experiences of others. In doing so, we not only honor our own journeys but also contribute to a larger narrative of compassion and understanding. Together, we can navigate the complexities of life and loss, finding solace in the connections we forge along the way. In the end, it is these connections that will sustain us, reminding us that we are all part of a shared human experience, bound together by our stories, our struggles, and our triumphs.

Chapter 8: The Role of Professional Care: Doctors, Nurses, and the Hospice Team

In the labyrinthine journey of life, particularly as one approaches its final chapters, the role of professional care becomes not just significant, but paramount. The medical professionals who navigate this terrain—doctors, nurses, and the dedicated hospice team—are not merely providers of care; they are the architects of dignity, comfort, and peace in a time that is often overshadowed by fear and uncertainty. Their expertise extends beyond the clinical; it encompasses the emotional, the psychological, and the spiritual dimensions of care. As we explore their roles, we must recognize that these professionals are not just tasked with managing symptoms or prolonging life; they are entrusted with the profound responsibility of guiding individuals and families through one of life's most challenging transitions.

To understand the impact of professional care, we must first appreciate the complexities of end-of-life experiences. Each person's journey is unique, shaped by their medical history, personal beliefs, and the relationships they hold dear. Here, the physician often serves as the first point of contact, tasked with not only diagnosing and prescribing but also with listening and understanding. It is a delicate balance: the need to convey medical realities while respecting the emotional landscape of the patient and their loved ones. The best physicians know that their role extends far beyond the clinical; they are advocates for the patient's wishes, interpreters of the medical labyrinth, and, at times, the bearers of difficult truths. They must navigate the fine line between hope and realism, helping patients and families to understand the implications of their choices while providing them with the support they need to make informed decisions.

Nurses, on the other hand, often become the heart of the healthcare team. Their presence is a constant throughout the chaotic whirlwind of hospital stays, home care, and hospice environments. Nurses are the ones who spend the most time with patients, observing the subtle shifts in their condition, their moods, and their needs. They are skilled not only in administering medications and managing pain but also in providing emotional support and companionship. In many ways, nurses are the unsung heroes of end-of-life care. They possess an innate ability to create a sense of safety and calm, often becoming the trusted confidants of patients and families alike. The power of a gentle touch, a reassuring word, or a moment of shared silence cannot be overstated. In the face of fear and uncertainty, nurses provide a steady presence, guiding families through the complexities of care and helping them to find moments of peace amidst the chaos.

The hospice team represents a holistic approach to end-of-life care, integrating a variety of disciplines to address the multifaceted needs of patients and their families. This interdisciplinary team typically includes not only doctors and nurses but also social workers, chaplains, and volunteers. Each member brings a unique perspective and set of skills, working collaboratively to ensure that the patient's physical, emotional, and spiritual needs are met. Social workers play a crucial role in navigating the practical aspects of care, helping families to access resources, manage logistics, and cope with the emotional weight of impending loss. They facilitate difficult conversations, guiding families through the decision-making process and helping them to articulate their wishes and fears. Chaplains, regardless of their specific religious affiliations, offer spiritual support, providing comfort and guidance to those grappling with existential questions and the search for meaning in the face of mortality.

The integration of these diverse roles underscores a fundamental truth: end-of-life care is not merely about the individual; it is about the family and the community as well. The hospice team recognizes that the experience of dying affects not just the patient but also their loved ones, who often find themselves navigating their own grief and uncertainty. By offering education, support, and resources, the hospice team empowers families to engage in the caregiving process, fostering an environment where love and connection can flourish even in the face of impending loss. This holistic approach is what distinguishes hospice care from traditional medical models; it emphasizes quality of life over quantity, prioritizing comfort and dignity as life draws to a close.

As we reflect on the role of professional care in the end-of-life journey, it is essential to acknowledge the emotional toll that this work can take on healthcare providers. The constant exposure to suffering and loss can lead to compassion fatigue, a phenomenon that can affect even the most dedicated professionals. It is vital for healthcare organizations to recognize this challenge and to provide support and resources for their staff. When caregivers are nurtured and supported, they are better equipped to provide compassionate care to their patients and families. This creates a virtuous cycle where the well-being of caregivers directly impacts the quality of care that patients receive.

In the context of professional care, communication emerges as a cornerstone of effective end-of-life support. The ability to engage in open, honest conversations about prognosis, treatment options, and personal wishes is essential. Yet, these conversations can be fraught with difficulty. Patients and families may struggle to articulate their fears and desires, while healthcare providers may grapple with how to convey complex medical information in a way that is both clear and compassionate. It is here that the role of active listening becomes critical. Healthcare providers must cultivate an environment where patients and families feel safe to express their thoughts and emotions. This requires not only technical expertise but also a deep sense of empathy and a willingness to engage in the emotional labor that accompanies end-of-life discussions.

Moreover, the importance of advanced care planning cannot be overstated. Professional caregivers play a crucial role in guiding patients and families through the process of articulating their values and preferences for end-of-life care. This involves discussions about the types of interventions that align with the patient's goals, as well as the potential benefits and burdens of various treatment options. By fostering these conversations early in the process, healthcare providers can help to ensure that patients receive care that is consistent with their wishes, thereby reducing the likelihood of distress and conflict later on. Advanced care planning is not a one-time event but an ongoing dialogue that evolves as circumstances change. It is a gift that patients can give to their loved ones, alleviating the burden of decision-making during an already challenging time.

As we navigate the complexities of end-of-life care, it is essential to recognize the profound impact that professional caregivers have on the overall experience of dying. Their expertise, compassion, and dedication can transform a potentially isolating and frightening journey into one that is characterized by connection, dignity, and peace. By embracing a holistic approach to care that addresses the physical, emotional, and spiritual dimensions of the end-of-life experience, healthcare professionals can create an environment where patients and families feel supported and empowered. In this way, the role of professional care transcends the clinical; it becomes a vital part of the human experience, reminding us of the importance of compassion, connection, and the shared journey of life and death.

In the end, the legacy of professional caregivers is not just found in the medical interventions they provide or the technical skills they possess. It lies in the moments of connection they create, the comfort they offer, and the respect they extend to every individual's unique journey. As we reflect on the role of these dedicated professionals, let us honor their commitment to fostering dignity and peace in the face of life's most profound challenges. In doing so, we can better appreciate the intricate web of care that surrounds us, reminding us that even in the darkest moments, we are never truly alone.

Chapter 9 - Caregiving Essentials: Compassion Without Burnout

In the intricate tapestry of life, caregiving often emerges as one of the most profound yet challenging roles one can assume. It is a journey marked by love, sacrifice, and an unwavering commitment to the well-being of another. Yet, as noble as this calling is, the reality of caregiving is fraught with emotional and physical demands that, if unaddressed, can lead to burnout. The essence of caregiving lies not only in the act of providing care but also in the manner in which caregivers nurture their own well-being amidst the demands placed upon them. The delicate balance between compassion for others and self-care is paramount, and recognizing this balance is the first step toward sustainable caregiving.

The emotional landscape of caregiving is often tumultuous. Caregivers frequently navigate a whirlwind of feelings—fear, anxiety, guilt, and even resentment can surface as they face the daily challenges of providing care. The person they love may be experiencing pain, confusion, or a decline in their health, and the caregiver is left to grapple with the reality of loss while simultaneously trying to provide comfort. This dual burden can be overwhelming. Caregivers may feel the weight of responsibility pressing down on them, fearing that any misstep could lead to further suffering for their loved one. This fear can spiral into a sense of inadequacy, leading caregivers to question their abilities and worth. It is crucial for caregivers to understand that these feelings are not only valid but also common. Acknowledging the emotional toll of caregiving is the first step in mitigating its effects.

Moreover, the physical demands of caregiving can be equally taxing. The daily tasks of assisting with personal hygiene, managing medications, and providing transportation to medical appointments can take a toll on the caregiver's body. Many caregivers neglect their own health in the process, often prioritizing their loved one's needs above their own. This neglect can manifest in various ways—chronic fatigue, sleep disturbances, and even physical ailments stemming from stress. The irony is that, in striving to be the best caregiver possible, they may inadvertently compromise their own health, which ultimately undermines their ability to provide care. It is a cycle that can be difficult to break, but it is essential for caregivers to recognize that their well-being is inextricably linked to the quality of care they provide. When caregivers take the time to rest, nourish themselves, and seek support, they not only enhance their own resilience but also improve the care they offer.

Establishing boundaries is another crucial aspect of sustainable caregiving. Many caregivers struggle with the notion of saying no, often feeling that they must be available at all times to meet their loved one's needs. However, this mindset can lead to exhaustion and resentment. Caregivers need to understand that it is acceptable to set limits on their availability, to carve out time for themselves, and to seek help when needed. This may involve enlisting the support of family members, friends, or professional caregivers who can share the burden. By creating a support network, caregivers can alleviate some of the pressures they face and allow themselves the space to recharge. It is important to remember that caregiving is not a solitary journey; it is a communal experience that thrives on collaboration and shared responsibility.

In the midst of caregiving, it is also vital to cultivate moments of joy and connection. The act of caring for someone can often overshadow the beauty of the relationship itself. Caregivers may find themselves so focused on the tasks at hand that they forget to engage with their loved one on a deeper level. Taking time to share stories, reminisce about fond memories, or simply enjoy a quiet moment together can infuse the caregiving experience with meaning and warmth. These moments serve as reminders of the love that binds caregivers and their loved ones, transforming the caregiving journey into one that is not solely defined by illness and hardship but also by love and connection.

Furthermore, caregivers should not hesitate to seek professional help when needed. Therapy or counseling can provide a safe space for caregivers to express their feelings, process their experiences, and develop coping strategies. Professional support can offer valuable perspectives and tools that empower caregivers to navigate their emotional landscape more effectively. Additionally, support groups can foster a sense of community, allowing caregivers to connect with others who understand their struggles. Sharing experiences, insights, and encouragement can be incredibly validating and can help alleviate the sense of isolation that often accompanies caregiving.

As caregivers navigate the complexities of their roles, it is essential to recognize the importance of self-compassion. Caregivers often hold themselves to impossibly high standards, believing that they must be perfect in their care. However, embracing the idea that it is okay to be imperfect can be liberating. Mistakes will happen, and there will be days when caregivers feel overwhelmed or inadequate. Acknowledging these moments without judgment allows caregivers to be kinder to themselves and fosters a healthier mindset. Practicing self-compassion involves treating oneself with the same kindness and understanding that one would offer to a dear friend in a similar situation. This shift in perspective can help caregivers cultivate resilience and sustain their capacity to care for others.

In the grander scheme of caregiving, it is essential to remember the significance of the journey itself. The act of caring for another human being is a profound expression of love, and it can lead to moments of deep connection and understanding. Caregivers often find that, in their efforts to support their loved ones, they also discover new facets of themselves. They may uncover strengths they never knew they possessed or develop a greater appreciation for the fragility of life. This journey can be transformative, leading to a deeper understanding of what it means to live fully—both for themselves and for those they care for.

Ultimately, the essence of caregiving lies in compassion—compassion for others and compassion for oneself. It is a delicate dance that requires balance, patience, and an unwavering commitment to well-being. By prioritizing self-care, establishing boundaries, and embracing the emotional complexities of the caregiving experience, caregivers can navigate this journey with grace and resilience. They can transform the challenges of caregiving into opportunities for growth, connection, and profound love. In doing so, they not only honor the lives of those they care for but also cultivate a richer, more meaningful existence for themselves. As we embark on this journey of life, loss, and love, let us remember that the path of caregiving is not only about giving but also about receiving—the gift of compassion, connection, and the shared human experience.

Chapter 10: Creating a Circle of Care: Family, Friends, and Community

In the intricate tapestry of life, the threads of connection form a vital fabric that supports us through the most challenging times. As we navigate the complexities of illness, loss, and the inevitable transitions that accompany them, the significance of a robust circle of care becomes unmistakably clear. This circle is not merely a network of relationships; it is a sanctuary, a source of strength, and a repository of love and compassion that can transform the experience of facing mortality into a journey marked by dignity and grace. The act of creating this circle is both a personal and communal endeavor, one that requires intention, vulnerability, and a willingness to reach out and embrace others.

When we think about care in the context of end-of-life experiences, it is easy to envision a sterile hospital room or a bustling hospice facility filled with medical professionals. However, true care extends far beyond the clinical setting. It encompasses the warmth of a friend's hand, the understanding gaze of a family member, and the collective presence of a community that rallies around an individual in need. This is where the essence of caregiving lies—not solely in the actions taken but in the relationships nurtured and the emotional bonds forged. In creating a circle of care, we are not just assembling a team of caregivers; we are cultivating a community that honors the human experience in all its complexity.

The journey begins with family. Family members often serve as the first line of support, providing comfort, companionship, and a sense of continuity in the face of change. However, the dynamics within families can be fraught with tension, unspoken grievances, and differing perspectives on how to provide care. In many cases, the stress of caregiving can exacerbate existing conflicts or create new ones. It is essential to approach these relationships with empathy and openness, recognizing that each person involved may be grappling with their own fears, uncertainties, and emotional responses. Open communication becomes a cornerstone of effective caregiving within families, allowing members to express their needs and concerns while fostering a collaborative approach to care.

Beyond family, friends play an indispensable role in creating a circle of care. They offer a different kind of support—one that is often less burdened by familial expectations and history. Friends can provide laughter, distraction, and a sense of normalcy amid the chaos of illness and loss. They can help lighten the emotional load, reminding us that joy can coexist with sorrow. However, it is crucial to recognize that not all friendships are equipped to handle the weight of caregiving. Some friends may feel uncomfortable or unsure of how to engage with someone facing serious illness. It is our responsibility to guide them, to articulate our needs and to invite them into our experiences. This invitation can take many forms, from simple requests for companionship to more specific asks, such as assistance with daily tasks or emotional support during difficult moments.

As we expand our circle of care, we must also consider the broader community. Neighbors, colleagues, and even acquaintances can contribute to the support network in meaningful ways. Community resources, such as local support groups, religious organizations, and volunteer services, can provide additional layers of assistance. Engaging with these resources not only alleviates some of the burdens of caregiving but also fosters a sense of belonging and connection. In many cultures, communal care is a deeply ingrained value, where the well-being of one is seen as a reflection of the well-being of all. Embracing this ethos can transform the experience of caregiving from an isolating endeavor into a collective journey, rich with shared experiences and mutual support.

Creating a circle of care also requires us to confront our own vulnerabilities. Accepting help can be a daunting task, especially for those who have prided themselves on their independence. The myths of self-sufficiency can create barriers that prevent us from reaching out to others. However, acknowledging our limitations and allowing ourselves to be supported is a powerful act of courage. It is an invitation for others to step into their roles as caregivers, allowing them to express their love and concern. In this exchange, we create a reciprocal relationship where giving and receiving become intertwined, enriching the lives of both the caregiver and the one receiving care.

Moreover, it is essential to recognize that the circle of care is not static; it evolves over time. As circumstances change, so too may the needs of the individual facing illness and the dynamics within the circle. Regular check-ins and open dialogues can help ensure that everyone involved feels valued and understood. It is also vital to be attuned to the emotional well-being of caregivers themselves. Caregiving can be demanding, often leading to burnout or compassion fatigue. By fostering an environment where caregivers can express their feelings and seek support, we reinforce the resilience of the entire circle.

In addition to emotional support, practical assistance is another critical component of a robust circle of care. This may include help with household chores, meal preparation, transportation to medical appointments, or even simple companionship during hospital stays. The act of providing practical help can alleviate some of the stress associated with caregiving, allowing both the caregiver and the individual receiving care to focus on what truly matters: the quality of the time spent together. Encouraging those in your circle to contribute in ways that align with their strengths and abilities can enhance the overall experience, creating a sense of purpose and fulfillment for all involved.

As we delve deeper into the concept of community in caregiving, we must also acknowledge the role of professional caregivers. While family and friends form the emotional backbone of a circle of care, trained professionals such as nurses, social workers, and hospice staff bring invaluable expertise and resources. They can help navigate the complexities of medical care, provide guidance on pain management, and offer emotional support to both the individual and their loved ones. Integrating professional care into the circle enhances the overall quality of support and ensures that the individual's needs are met holistically.

Ultimately, creating a circle of care is about fostering a sense of belonging and connection. It is about recognizing that we are not alone in our struggles and that there is strength in vulnerability. As we open ourselves to the support of others, we create a space where love, compassion, and understanding can flourish. This circle becomes a testament to the power of human connection, reminding us that even in the face of life's most profound challenges, we have the capacity to find solace in one another.

In conclusion, the journey of caregiving is not one that should be undertaken in isolation. It is a shared experience, a dance of give and take that enriches the lives of everyone involved. By intentionally creating a circle of care that encompasses family, friends, and community, we can navigate the complexities of illness and loss with greater resilience and grace. This circle becomes a source of strength, a reminder that we are all interconnected and that together, we can face the inevitable transitions of life with dignity and love. As we lean on each other, we not only honor the journey of those we care for but also enrich our own lives in the process, creating a legacy of compassion that transcends the boundaries of time and circumstance.

Chapter 11: Coping with Terminal Diagnoses: A Path Forward

Receiving a terminal diagnosis is a moment that forever alters the landscape of existence. It marks a profound shift in the narrative of life, a jarring interruption of what was once a predictable, albeit imperfect, journey. The news often feels like a seismic event, shattering the illusion of control and certainty that many of us cling to. In that instant, the future is no longer a blank canvas filled with possibilities; instead, it becomes a stark, unyielding reality, painted in shades of fear, uncertainty, and profound sadness. Yet, within this darkened space, there exists the potential for transformation, for a redefinition of what it means to live fully in the face of mortality.

The initial response to a terminal diagnosis can vary

widely from person to person. For some, it is a rush of disbelief, a protective mechanism that momentarily shields them from the weight of the truth. "This can't be happening to me," they might think, as if sheer will could rewrite their fate. Others may plunge into despair, grappling with the enormity of the loss that looms ahead. In these moments, it is essential to acknowledge the multitude of emotions that arise—fear, anger, sadness, and even moments of clarity or acceptance. Each of these feelings is a natural part of the human experience, a testament to the depth of our connections and the richness of our lives.

As the initial shock begins to fade, the reality of the diagnosis sets in. It is here that the journey toward coping truly begins. This journey is not linear; it is a winding path filled with detours and unexpected turns. One of the first steps on this path is the need to process the diagnosis and its implications. This can involve engaging in conversations with healthcare providers, seeking clarity about the illness, and understanding the options available for treatment and care. Knowledge can be empowering, providing a sense of agency in a situation that often feels disempowering. It is crucial to ask questions, to seek out information, and to involve loved ones in these discussions, creating a support system that will prove invaluable as the journey unfolds.

In the face of a terminal diagnosis, establishing a sense of purpose becomes paramount. What does it mean to live fully when time is limited? For many, this question prompts a reevaluation of priorities, a shedding of the trivial in favor of what truly matters. Relationships often take center stage, and the desire to connect with family and friends deepens. It is a time for vulnerability, for sharing fears and hopes, for expressing love and gratitude. The act of reaching out can be profoundly healing, transforming the isolation that often accompanies illness into a shared experience of humanity.

However, the path of coping is not solely about connection with others; it also involves an inward journey. Reflection becomes a powerful tool in navigating the emotional landscape of terminal illness. Journaling, art, or simply quiet contemplation can help individuals articulate their feelings, fears, and desires. This process of self-exploration can illuminate what is truly significant, guiding decisions about how to spend the remaining time. Some may find solace in revisiting cherished memories, while others may seek to create new experiences, whether through travel, family gatherings, or quiet moments of beauty in nature.

As the diagnosis permeates daily life, it is essential to cultivate a mindset that embraces the present. Mindfulness practices can offer a refuge from the storm of anxiety about the future. Grounding oneself in the here and now can reveal moments of joy, even amid sorrow. A warm cup of tea, the laughter of a grandchild, the beauty of a sunset—these seemingly small experiences can become profound reminders of life's richness. It is through this lens of presence that individuals can begin to find meaning, even in the face of impending loss.

Navigating a terminal diagnosis also requires a shift in how we perceive hope. Hope does not always equate to a cure; it can manifest in many forms. For some, it may mean hoping for quality of life, for pain-free days, or for the opportunity to say goodbye in a meaningful way. Others may find hope in the legacy they wish to leave behind or in the relationships they nurture. This reframing of hope can bring comfort and strength, allowing individuals to face each day with intention and purpose.

In the midst of this journey, it is crucial to recognize the role of professional support. The healthcare team—doctors, nurses, social workers, and hospice providers—can offer invaluable guidance and resources. They are trained not only to address the physical aspects of illness but also to provide emotional and spiritual support. Engaging with these professionals can help individuals and families navigate the complexities of care, making informed decisions that align with their values and wishes. Hospice care, in particular, emphasizes comfort and dignity, allowing individuals to spend their remaining time in a manner that honors their preferences and priorities.

As the journey progresses, the reality of mortality becomes increasingly tangible. It is a time for difficult conversations, for discussing end-of-life wishes, and for making plans that reflect one's values. These discussions can be daunting, often fraught with discomfort and fear. Yet, they are essential in ensuring that individuals receive the care they desire and that their wishes are respected. It is an act of love, a way to alleviate the burden on loved ones who may otherwise be left to make decisions in the absence of guidance.

As individuals approach the end of life, the concept of legacy often emerges as a focal point. What do we wish to be remembered for? How can we ensure that our values and beliefs endure beyond our physical presence? This contemplation can lead to meaningful actions, whether through storytelling, creating art, or engaging in projects that reflect one's passions. The act of leaving a legacy can be profoundly fulfilling, transforming the focus from loss to the celebration of a life well-lived.

Coping with a terminal diagnosis is undeniably challenging, yet it also offers a unique opportunity for growth and connection. It is a journey that compels individuals to confront their fears, to embrace vulnerability, and to seek out the beauty that exists even in the shadow of death. In this space, we discover the profound truth that life, in all its complexity, is a gift to be cherished. Each moment, each interaction, and each breath becomes imbued with meaning, urging us to live fully until the very end. Through this lens, we can find a path forward—a way to navigate the uncharted waters of mortality with grace, compassion, and an unwavering commitment to the richness of the human experience.

Chapter 12 - Grief as a Journey: From Denial to Acceptance

Grief is often portrayed as a linear process, a neat progression from one stage to the next, each phase clearly defined and easily identifiable. However, the reality is far more complex and nuanced. Grief is not a straight path but rather a winding journey, filled with unexpected detours and uncharted territories. It is a deeply personal experience, shaped by our relationships, our histories, and our individual responses to loss. When we confront the death of a loved one, we are thrust into a landscape of emotions that can feel overwhelming and chaotic. Denial may be our first instinct, a protective mechanism shielding us from the rawness of our pain. It is a natural response, a way to create a buffer against the shock of loss. We may find ourselves going through the motions of daily life, acting as if nothing has changed, even while a profound absence looms large in our hearts. This denial can be comforting for a time, allowing us to maintain a semblance of normalcy as we grapple with the reality of what has happened. Yet, as the days turn into weeks and the weeks into months, the truth begins to seep through the cracks of our defenses. The weight of our sorrow becomes impossible to ignore, and we are forced to confront the reality of our grief.

As we move beyond denial, we may encounter a tumultuous wave of emotions: anger, guilt, sadness, and confusion. Each feeling can hit us like a tidal wave, pulling us under and leaving us gasping for air. Anger may surface as we grapple with the unfairness of our loss, questioning why it happened and why it happened to us. We may feel anger towards the person who has died, towards ourselves for not being able to save them, or towards the world for continuing on as if nothing has changed. This anger can be a double-edged sword; while it can fuel our desire for answers and justice, it can also isolate us from those around us, creating a barrier that prevents connection and understanding. Guilt often accompanies anger, a nagging voice that whispers we could have done more, been better, or somehow altered the course of events. This guilt can be paralyzing, trapping us in a cycle of self-blame that hinders our healing. It is essential to recognize that these feelings are a normal part of the grieving process. They do not define us, nor do they diminish the love we had for the person we lost. Instead, they are markers on our journey, signposts that remind us of the depth of our connection and the magnitude of our loss.

As we navigate this emotional landscape, we may find ourselves fluctuating between these feelings, sometimes experiencing them all in a single day. One moment we may feel a surge of anger, and the next, a wave of profound sadness. This ebb and flow can be disorienting, leaving us unsure of where we stand or how to move forward. It is crucial to allow ourselves the space to feel these emotions fully, to acknowledge them without judgment. Grief is not something to be rushed through or avoided; it is an experience to be lived and embraced. In doing so, we honor our loved ones and the impact they had on our lives. As we journey deeper into our grief, we may encounter moments of clarity and insight. These moments can be fleeting, but they often provide a glimpse of the healing that is possible. We may find ourselves reflecting on the memories we shared, the lessons learned, and the love that continues to exist despite the physical absence of our loved one. These reflections can serve as anchors, grounding us amidst the storm of our emotions. They remind us that while our loved one may no longer be with us in body, their spirit and influence remain a part of our lives.

Acceptance, the final stage of grief, is often misunderstood. It is not a destination we reach after traversing the landscape of denial, anger, and sadness; rather, it is a continual process of coming to terms with our loss.

Acceptance does not mean we no longer feel pain or miss the person we lost. Instead, it signifies a shift in our relationship with that pain. We begin to integrate our grief into our lives, allowing it to coexist with our memories and our love. We learn to carry our loss with us, rather than allowing it to define us. This process of acceptance can be gradual, often requiring us to confront our feelings repeatedly. It may involve revisiting memories, celebrating milestones, and acknowledging the void left behind. It may also necessitate a reevaluation of our own lives, as we consider how we want to move forward in the wake of our loss. As we embrace acceptance, we may find ourselves discovering new ways to honor our loved ones. This could take the form of rituals, such as lighting a candle on anniversaries or creating a scrapbook filled with cherished memories. It may also involve finding ways to give back to the community or supporting causes that were important to our loved ones. In these acts of remembrance, we not only keep their memory alive but also create a legacy that reflects their values and spirit.

Ultimately, the journey of grief is one of transformation. It challenges us to confront our deepest fears and vulnerabilities, forcing us to reevaluate our relationships and our understanding of love and loss. While the path may be fraught with pain, it can also lead to profound insights and a greater appreciation for the fragility of life. As we learn to navigate our grief, we may find ourselves more attuned to the beauty and complexity of our emotions, more compassionate towards ourselves and others, and more open to the possibility of joy amidst sorrow. In this way, grief becomes not just a burden to bear but a powerful teacher, guiding us toward a deeper understanding of what it means to live fully. In the end, the journey through grief is not about forgetting our loved ones or moving on from our loss; it is about finding a way to carry them with us as we continue to navigate the ever-changing landscape of our lives. It is about learning to live in a world where their absence is felt but not defined. It is a journey that requires patience, resilience, and a willingness to embrace the complexities of our emotions. As we walk this path, we may discover that grief, while painful, is also a testament to the love we shared and the impact our loved ones had on our lives. It is a journey that ultimately leads us toward acceptance, healing, and a renewed sense of purpose as we learn to live fully, even in the face of loss.

Chapter 13 - Emotional Healing: Finding Peace Amid Loss

In the wake of loss, the emotional landscape can feel like a vast, uncharted territory, filled with both familiar and foreign terrains of grief. It is a journey that each of us must navigate in our own way, often marked by a series of waves that ebb and flow, sometimes crashing violently upon the shores of our hearts, and at other times retreating to reveal moments of calm. The depth of emotional healing is not merely about the absence of pain; rather, it is about the transformation of that pain into something that can coexist with the memory of love and the essence of those we have lost. This process is as unique as the individual experiencing it, shaped by our relationships, our histories, and our capacity to find meaning amid the chaos.

When we lose someone we cherish, the initial response is often a profound sense of dislocation. The world, once vibrant and full of possibilities, can suddenly feel dimmed, as if a veil has been drawn over our perception. Familiar routines become laden with reminders of absence, and the simple act of moving through a day can feel like an insurmountable challenge. It is in this disorientation that we begin to grapple with the myriad emotions that accompany grief: sadness, anger, confusion, and sometimes even guilt. Each of these feelings is a thread in the intricate tapestry of our experience, and while they may seem overwhelming at first, they are essential to the process of healing. Acknowledging these emotions is the first step toward understanding them, allowing us to transform our grief from a burden into a catalyst for growth.

As we embark on this journey of emotional healing, the importance of self-compassion cannot be overstated. In a society that often prizes stoicism and self-sufficiency, we may feel pressured to suppress our emotions or to "move on" before we are ready. Yet, healing is not a linear process; it is a winding path that requires us to honor our feelings, no matter how uncomfortable they may be. Embracing vulnerability allows us to experience the full spectrum of our emotions, providing a fertile ground for healing to take root. When we permit ourselves to grieve openly, we create space for our emotions to breathe, for our hearts to mend, and for our souls to begin the work of reconciling loss with love.

In the midst of grief, we often find ourselves yearning for connection. The presence of others can be a balm for our wounds, reminding us that we are not alone in our suffering. Reaching out to friends and family, sharing stories, and recalling moments spent with our loved ones can foster a sense of community that is essential for healing. These connections serve as lifelines, anchoring us in the present while honoring the past. In this shared space, we can find solace in knowing that our grief is valid and that others bear witness to our pain. It is through these interactions that we begin to weave our memories into the fabric of our lives, allowing them to coexist with our ongoing journey.

Yet, the process of healing is not solely reliant on our relationships with others; it also requires introspection and self-discovery. Journaling, meditation, and creative expression can serve as powerful tools for processing our emotions and finding clarity amid the turmoil. By putting pen to paper or engaging in artistic endeavors, we create an opportunity to explore our inner landscapes, giving voice to thoughts and feelings that may otherwise remain trapped within. This act of creation can be cathartic, allowing us to externalize our grief and transform it into something tangible, something that can be understood and shared. In the quiet moments of reflection, we may discover insights that illuminate our path forward, guiding us toward a deeper understanding of ourselves and our relationship with loss.

As we navigate the complexities of emotional healing, we may also encounter the notion of meaning-making. In the aftermath of loss, we often find ourselves grappling with existential questions: What does it mean to live fully in the face of mortality? How do we honor the legacy of those we have lost? These questions can feel daunting, yet they also present an opportunity for profound growth. By seeking to understand the significance of our loved ones' lives and the impact they had on our own, we can begin to weave their memory into our ongoing narrative. This process of meaning-making allows us to reframe our grief, transforming it from a source of despair into a testament to love and connection.

In the context of emotional healing, rituals can play a vital role. Whether it is lighting a candle on the anniversary of a loved one's passing, creating a memory box filled with cherished mementos, or participating in a community gathering to celebrate their life, these acts can provide a sense of continuity and connection. Rituals help us to honor our grief while also acknowledging the enduring presence of our loved ones in our lives. They serve as a bridge between the past and the present, allowing us to carry forward the essence of those we have lost while also embracing the possibilities of the future. In this way, healing becomes not just an individual journey, but a collective one, rooted in shared experiences and communal support.

As we continue to explore the terrain of loss, it is essential to recognize that healing does not imply forgetting. Instead, it is about finding a way to integrate our grief into the tapestry of our lives. The memories of our loved ones can become guiding stars, illuminating our paths and reminding us of the values and lessons they imparted. In this integration, we may discover new ways to honor their legacy, whether through acts of kindness, advocacy, or simply by living authentically in a way that reflects their influence. The love we shared does not diminish with loss; rather, it transforms, becoming a source of strength and inspiration as we navigate the complexities of life without them.

In moments of quiet reflection, we may find ourselves contemplating the nature of love itself. Love is not bound by time or space; it transcends the physical realm, weaving itself into the very fabric of our being. The love we shared with those we have lost continues to exist, shaping our thoughts, actions, and emotions. It is this enduring connection that can provide solace in our darkest moments, reminding us that while our loved ones may no longer be present in body, their spirit lives on within us. As we move forward, we can carry their love as a guiding light, illuminating our path and infusing our lives with purpose and meaning.

Ultimately, the journey of emotional healing is one of transformation. It is a process that allows us to emerge from the depths of grief with a renewed sense of self, a deeper understanding of our capacity for love, and a greater appreciation for the fragility and beauty of life. In this transformation, we may find that our experiences of loss have equipped us with a profound empathy for others who are navigating similar paths. We become bearers of wisdom, able to offer support and understanding to those who are grappling with their own grief. In this way, our healing becomes a gift that we can share with the world, fostering connection and compassion in a society that often struggles to confront the realities of loss.

As we embrace the complexities of our emotions and the richness of our memories, we can begin to forge a new relationship with our grief—one that honors the past while also embracing the present. This journey is not about erasing the pain of loss, but rather about finding peace amid it. It is about learning to live fully, with our hearts open to both joy and sorrow, and recognizing that in every chapter of our lives, there is an opportunity for healing, connection, and ultimately, love. In this delicate dance between loss and love, we discover the resilience of the human spirit, the capacity to find beauty in the midst of sorrow, and the profound truth that even in our darkest moments, we are never truly alone.

Chapter 14 - Confronting Fear: The Courage to Face Mortality

Fear is a powerful emotion, one that can grip us tightly and hold us in a state of paralysis. It is an emotion that is often whispered about in the quiet corners of our minds but rarely spoken aloud. Fear of the unknown, fear of pain, fear of loss, and ultimately, fear of death itself. In the context of end-of-life choices, this fear can be magnified, becoming a formidable barrier that hinders our ability to engage with the reality of our mortality. Yet, confronting this fear is not only essential for those facing their own end-of-life journey but also for caregivers, family members, and friends who share in this experience. It is through this confrontation that we can begin to find a sense of peace and acceptance.

The first step in confronting fear is recognizing its presence. Much like a shadow, fear can loom large and distort our perceptions. It can manifest in various forms: anxiety about what lies ahead, dread of suffering, or the overwhelming sadness of saying goodbye. For many, this fear is compounded by societal taboos surrounding death and dying. We live in a culture that often avoids discussions about mortality, relegating them to hushed conversations or the confines of a therapist's office. This avoidance can lead to a sense of isolation, as individuals grappling with these fears feel they must navigate their emotions alone. Yet, it is crucial to understand that fear is a universal experience. Acknowledging this can help us to feel less isolated and more connected to others who share similar anxieties.

Once we recognize our fears, the next step is to explore their roots. What is it that we truly fear? Is it the physical pain associated with dying? The emotional turmoil of leaving loved ones behind? Or perhaps the fear of not having lived fully? By delving into these questions, we can begin to unpack the complexities of our emotions. It is often said that knowledge is power, and in this context, understanding our fears can empower us to confront them head-on. For instance, if the fear of pain is at the forefront, seeking information about palliative care or hospice services can provide reassurance. Knowing that there are options available to manage pain and ensure comfort can alleviate some of that fear and allow for a more peaceful acceptance of the inevitable.

In my work as a physician, I have witnessed firsthand the transformative power of open conversations about death. When patients and their families are willing to engage in these discussions, fears can be addressed and demystified. It is not uncommon for individuals to express their fears about dying alone or in pain. However, when they learn about the support systems available—such as hospice care, which focuses on providing comfort and dignity in the final stages of life—they often find solace. The fear of the unknown begins to dissipate, replaced by a sense of agency and control over their circumstances. This shift can be profound, allowing individuals to embrace their mortality with a newfound sense of courage.

In confronting fear, it is also essential to cultivate a mindset of acceptance. Acceptance does not mean resignation; rather, it is an acknowledgment of the reality of our situation. It is the recognition that life is finite and that death is a natural part of the human experience. This acceptance can be liberating, allowing us to focus on what truly matters in our remaining time. For many, this means prioritizing relationships, engaging in meaningful activities, and expressing love and gratitude to those around them. The fear of death can serve as a catalyst for living more fully, prompting us to examine our values and make choices that align with them.

Moreover, confronting fear can foster resilience. As we face our mortality, we often discover inner strengths and resources we did not know we possessed. This resilience can manifest in various ways, from the courage to have difficult conversations with loved ones to the determination to create a legacy that reflects our values. I have seen patients transform their fear into a desire to leave behind something meaningful, whether through storytelling, art, or acts of kindness. This shift in perspective can not only empower individuals but also inspire those around them to embrace their own journeys with courage and authenticity.

It is also important to remember that confronting fear is not a solitary endeavor. It is a collective experience that can be shared with loved ones, caregivers, and healthcare professionals. Creating a supportive environment where fears can be expressed and discussed openly can foster deeper connections and understanding. For families navigating the complexities of end-of-life care, this shared vulnerability can strengthen bonds and create a sense of unity in the face of adversity. It is a reminder that we are not alone in our fears; we are part of a larger tapestry of human experience, woven together by our shared struggles and triumphs.

As we confront fear, we must also be mindful of the language we use. Words hold power, and the way we speak about death can influence our perceptions and emotions. Instead of framing death as a defeat or an end, we can choose to view it as a transition—a natural progression in the cycle of life. This shift in language can help to reframe our fears and allow us to approach the topic of mortality with greater compassion and understanding. It is an invitation to engage in conversations that honor the complexity of our emotions while also celebrating the beauty of life.

In the end, confronting fear is an act of courage. It requires vulnerability, honesty, and a willingness to engage with the uncomfortable. Yet, it is through this confrontation that we can find peace amid uncertainty. By acknowledging our fears and seeking to understand them, we can transform our relationship with mortality. We can cultivate resilience, deepen our connections with others, and ultimately embrace the fullness of life, even as we prepare for its inevitable conclusion. In doing so, we honor not only our own journeys but also the journeys of those we love, creating a legacy of courage and compassion that extends far beyond our final days. As we navigate the complexities of life, loss, and the journey to peace, let us remember that it is in facing our fears that we truly learn to live fully.

Chapter 15: Spiritual and Emotional Comfort: The Search for Inner Peace

In the quiet moments of our lives, when the cacophony of daily existence fades, we often find ourselves grappling with deeper questions about purpose, connection, and the essence of our being. As we navigate the complexities of life, especially in the face of illness and impending loss, the pursuit of spiritual and emotional comfort becomes paramount. It is in these moments of vulnerability that we may discover the profound depths of our own humanity, and the rich tapestry of relationships that have shaped our journey. The search for inner peace is not merely an abstract concept; it is a tangible quest that can guide us through the tumultuous waters of grief, fear, and uncertainty.

Spiritual comfort can take many forms, often shaped by our individual beliefs, traditions, and experiences. For some, it may be rooted in organized religion, a set of doctrines that provide a framework for understanding the mysteries of life and death. For others, spirituality may be more fluid, encompassing a connection to nature, to art, or to the universe itself. Regardless of its manifestation, the essence of spiritual comfort lies in its ability to foster a sense of belonging and purpose, even in the face of mortality. It encourages us to reflect on our values, to seek meaning in our experiences, and to cultivate a sense of gratitude for the moments we have shared with others.

As we confront the realities of terminal illness, the importance of spiritual comfort becomes even more pronounced. It offers a refuge from the chaos of medical interventions and the anxiety of what lies ahead. Engaging in spiritual practices—whether through prayer, meditation, or simply spending time in nature—can provide a sense of grounding, a reminder that we are part of something larger than ourselves. In these moments, we may find solace in the rituals that have been passed down through generations, connecting us to our ancestors and to the collective human experience. These practices can serve as a balm for our souls, allowing us to confront our fears and uncertainties with grace and dignity.

Emotional comfort, on the other hand, often hinges on our relationships with those around us. The bonds we forge with family, friends, and caregivers can be a source of immense strength during times of crisis. In the face of loss, it is the love and support of others that can help us navigate the emotional landscape of grief. It is essential to cultivate these connections, to reach out and share our feelings, our fears, and our hopes. In doing so, we not only allow ourselves to be vulnerable but also invite others into our experience, creating a shared space of understanding and compassion. This reciprocal exchange can lead to profound healing, as we realize that we are not alone in our struggles.

The act of sharing our stories—our joys, our sorrows, our triumphs, and our defeats—can be a powerful tool for emotional comfort. In recounting our experiences, we weave a narrative that gives shape to our lives, helping us to make sense of the chaos that often accompanies loss. Storytelling can be a means of processing grief, allowing us to explore the complexities of our emotions in a safe and supportive environment. Whether through conversations with loved ones, journaling, or engaging in creative expression, the act of storytelling can illuminate the path toward healing, fostering a sense of connection and understanding.

In this journey toward inner peace, it is also crucial to acknowledge the role of self-compassion. As we face the realities of life and death, we may find ourselves grappling with feelings of guilt, regret, or inadequacy. It is all too easy to become consumed by the weight of these emotions, to allow them to cloud our judgment and hinder our ability to find solace. Practicing self-compassion involves treating ourselves with the same kindness and understanding that we would offer to a dear friend. It means recognizing that we are human, that we are fallible, and that our experiences—both positive and negative—are part of the rich tapestry of life. By embracing self-compassion, we open the door to healing, allowing ourselves to experience the full spectrum of our emotions without judgment.

As we seek spiritual and emotional comfort, it is essential to remain open to the myriad ways in which peace can manifest. For some, it may come in the form of quiet reflection during a sunset, while for others, it may be found in the laughter shared with loved ones. The key is to remain attuned to our own needs, to listen to the whispers of our hearts, and to honor the journey that is uniquely ours. This requires patience and practice, as we learn to navigate the complexities of our emotions and the intricacies of our relationships.

In the context of caregiving, both for ourselves and for others, the search for spiritual and emotional comfort can take on additional layers of significance. Caregivers often find themselves in a position of profound responsibility, balancing the needs of their loved ones with their own emotional well-being. It is crucial for caregivers to prioritize their own spiritual and emotional health, to seek out the support they need to sustain their own journeys. This may involve creating spaces for self-care, engaging in spiritual practices, or simply allowing themselves to grieve the losses they experience along the way. By nurturing their own spirits, caregivers can cultivate the resilience needed to provide compassionate care to others.

As we navigate the end-of-life journey, the importance of spiritual and emotional comfort cannot be overstated. It is in this space that we can confront our fears, embrace our vulnerability, and ultimately find peace in the face of uncertainty. The search for inner peace is a deeply personal journey, one that requires us to be honest with ourselves and with those we love. It invites us to explore the depths of our own souls, to seek out the connections that bring us joy, and to cultivate a sense of gratitude for the moments we have shared.

In the end, the quest for spiritual and emotional comfort is not merely about finding solace in the face of loss; it is about embracing the fullness of life itself. It is about recognizing that even in our darkest moments, there is beauty to be found, connections to be cherished, and lessons to be learned. As we embark on this journey, may we find the courage to seek out the comforts that resonate with our souls, and may we emerge from the shadows of grief with a renewed sense of purpose and peace. The journey toward inner peace is not a destination but an ongoing process, one that invites us to live fully in each moment, to honor our experiences, and to embrace the richness of the human experience.

Chapter 16: Palliative Care: Prioritizing Comfort and Quality of Life

In the landscape of healthcare, palliative care emerges as a compassionate bridge between the relentless pursuit of cure and the profound need for comfort. It is a realm where the focus shifts from aggressive treatments to the holistic well-being of the individual. For many, the word "palliative" conjures images of finality, yet it is a concept that should be embraced much earlier in the trajectory of illness. It is not solely about end-of-life care; rather, it is a philosophy that prioritizes quality of life, regardless of the stage of disease. The essence of palliative care lies in its recognition that living well is as critical as surviving. This chapter endeavors to illuminate the principles of palliative care, its profound impact on patients and families, and the transformative power it holds in navigating the complexities of serious illness.

At its core, palliative care is about understanding the individual as a whole person, rather than reducing them to their diagnosis. It acknowledges the intricate tapestry of emotions, relationships, and experiences that define a person's existence. This approach is particularly vital for those facing life-limiting illnesses, where the burden of symptoms can overshadow the richness of life itself. Pain management, emotional support, and spiritual care are woven into the fabric of palliative care, creating a comprehensive support system that honors the dignity of each individual. It is a reminder that even in the face of adversity, there exists the potential for joy, connection, and fulfillment.

One of the most significant aspects of palliative care is its emphasis on communication. Open dialogue between healthcare providers, patients, and families fosters an environment where fears and hopes can be shared openly. It is in these conversations that the true essence of palliative care is revealed—the understanding that patients have unique values and preferences that must guide their care. In a world where medical jargon can often obscure the human experience, palliative care practitioners strive to demystify the complexities of illness, ensuring that patients and their loved ones are active participants in their care decisions. This collaborative approach not only empowers patients but also cultivates a sense of agency in a time when they may feel most vulnerable.

Moreover, palliative care extends its reach beyond the confines of the hospital or clinic. It permeates the home, where many individuals prefer to spend their final days. Home-based palliative care teams provide invaluable support, allowing patients to remain in familiar surroundings, surrounded by loved ones. This model of care recognizes that the home is not just a physical space; it is a sanctuary that holds memories, comfort, and love. The ability to receive care in this environment can significantly enhance a patient's sense of control and emotional well-being. It is a testament to the belief that comfort can be found in the most intimate of settings, where the warmth of family and the echoes of laughter can coexist with the realities of illness.

As we delve deeper into the principles of palliative care, we encounter the essential element of symptom management. Pain, nausea, breathlessness—these are but a few of the myriad symptoms that can plague individuals with serious illnesses. Palliative care practitioners are trained to address these symptoms with precision and compassion, employing a variety of interventions tailored to the unique needs of each patient. This aspect of care is not merely about alleviating physical discomfort; it is about restoring a sense of normalcy and allowing individuals to engage in the activities that bring them joy. Whether it is savoring a favorite meal, enjoying a sunset, or spending quality time with family, the goal is to enhance the overall quality of life, even in the face of profound challenges.

The integration of psychological and emotional support is another cornerstone of palliative care. The emotional landscape of serious illness is often fraught with anxiety, fear, and uncertainty. Palliative care teams include social workers, psychologists, and chaplains who work collaboratively to address the emotional and spiritual dimensions of illness. This multifaceted approach recognizes that mental well-being is intricately linked to physical health. By providing a safe space for patients and families to express their fears and concerns, palliative care fosters resilience and coping strategies that can significantly improve the overall experience of illness. It is an affirmation that vulnerability is not a weakness, but rather a testament to the human spirit's capacity to endure and thrive, even in the face of adversity.

In addition to addressing the needs of the patient, palliative care extends its compassionate embrace to families. The impact of serious illness ripples through the family unit, often leaving loved ones grappling with their own fears and grief. Palliative care teams recognize that caregivers require support and respite, as they navigate the challenges of caring for someone with a serious illness. By providing education, resources, and emotional support, palliative care empowers families to be active participants in the caregiving process while also prioritizing their own well-being. This holistic approach acknowledges that the journey of illness is not a solitary one; it is a shared experience that requires the strength and resilience of both the patient and their loved ones.

As we reflect on the principles of palliative care, it becomes evident that this approach is not limited to those at the end of life. It is a philosophy that can and should be integrated into the care of individuals facing serious illnesses from the moment of diagnosis. The earlier palliative care is introduced, the more profound its impact can be. It is a proactive approach that seeks to prevent suffering before it becomes overwhelming. By addressing the physical, emotional, and spiritual dimensions of illness early on, palliative care can enhance the overall experience of patients and families, allowing them to navigate the complexities of illness with dignity and grace.

In a healthcare landscape often characterized by fragmentation and specialization, palliative care stands out as a beacon of holistic care. It is a reminder that at the heart of medicine lies the sacred duty to care for the whole person. As we continue to explore the intricacies of palliative care, we must advocate for its integration into the broader healthcare system, ensuring that every individual facing serious illness has access to the support and resources they need to live fully, even in the face of challenges. The journey through illness is not merely a passage toward death; it is an opportunity to embrace life's richness, to find meaning in every moment, and to prioritize comfort and quality of life above all else.

Ultimately, palliative care invites us to reconsider our relationship with illness and mortality. It challenges the notion that suffering is an inevitable part of the journey and instead offers a framework for finding peace amid uncertainty. By prioritizing comfort, dignity, and emotional well-being, palliative care transforms the experience of serious illness from one of despair to one of hope and resilience. It is a call to action for healthcare providers, patients, and families alike to embrace a new narrative—one that honors the complexity of human experience and affirms the beauty of living fully, even in the face of life's most profound challenges. In this journey toward understanding and acceptance, we find the courage to face the unknown, the strength to seek help, and the grace to navigate the intricate dance of life and loss with compassion and love.

Chapter 17: Hospice Care: A Compassionate Alternative to Prolonging Pain

In the quiet corridors of hospice care, there exists a profound understanding of life and death that transcends the clinical and ventures into the deeply human. Here, the focus shifts from the relentless pursuit of cure to the tender art of comfort. It is a space where the complexities of illness are met with compassion, where every breath is acknowledged as a testament to the life lived, and where the shadows of fear and uncertainty are softened by the presence of understanding. Hospice care embodies a philosophy that recognizes the inherent dignity of individuals facing the end of their lives. It invites us to reframe our perceptions of death, not as a failure of medicine, but as a natural progression of life—a transition that deserves to be met with grace and respect.

The essence of hospice care lies in its holistic approach, addressing not only the physical symptoms of illness but also the emotional, spiritual, and social dimensions of the dying process. Patients are not merely recipients of medical interventions; they are individuals with stories, relationships, and dreams that deserve recognition and honor. This perspective is vital, as it acknowledges that the experience of dying is as much about the quality of life as it is about the quantity of time left. In hospice, the emphasis is placed on living fully, even in the face of impending death—a concept that can be both liberating and transformative. Care teams work diligently to create an environment where patients can express their fears, share their hopes, and find moments of joy amidst the challenges they face.

A significant aspect of hospice care is its commitment to symptom management. Pain, nausea, anxiety, and other distressing symptoms can overshadow the final days of life, robbing individuals of the peace they deserve. Through a combination of medications, therapies, and supportive interventions, hospice teams strive to alleviate suffering and enhance comfort. This process is not merely about eliminating pain; it involves understanding the unique needs of each patient and tailoring care to their specific circumstances. The goal is to empower individuals to engage with their loved ones, to savor the simple pleasures of life, and to find solace in their surroundings. In this way, hospice becomes a sanctuary, a haven where the burdens of illness are eased, and the beauty of existence is celebrated.

Moreover, hospice care extends its reach beyond the patient to encompass the family and caregivers, recognizing that the experience of dying affects everyone involved. Family members often grapple with their own fears, guilt, and grief as they navigate the complexities of their loved one's illness. Hospice teams provide education, support, and counseling to help families cope with the emotional toll of caregiving and loss. This holistic approach fosters a sense of community, where individuals can share their experiences, find solace in one another, and cultivate resilience in the face of adversity. The bonds formed in these moments of vulnerability can be profound, creating a shared understanding of the fragility of life and the importance of cherishing every moment.

As we consider the philosophy of hospice care, it becomes clear that it is not solely about the act of dying, but rather about the art of living—living fully until the very end. This perspective challenges societal norms that often equate death with failure, urging us to embrace the inevitability of mortality with open hearts. In hospice, we are reminded that every moment is an opportunity for connection, reflection, and love. Whether it is a gentle hand squeeze, a shared laugh, or a quiet moment of understanding, these interactions become sacred experiences that enrich the lives of both patients and their families. The beauty of hospice care lies in its ability to create space for these moments, allowing individuals to express their emotions, share their stories, and find closure in their relationships.

In the context of hospice, difficult conversations about death and dying are not avoided but embraced. Care teams encourage open dialogue, providing patients and families with the opportunity to articulate their wishes, fears, and hopes. This process can be challenging, as it requires vulnerability and honesty. However, it is through these conversations that individuals can find clarity and peace. When patients are empowered to express their desires for their final days, they reclaim agency over their lives and deaths. They can articulate what matters most to them—whether it be spending time with loved ones, experiencing meaningful rituals, or simply enjoying the beauty of nature. In this way, hospice care becomes a collaborative journey, where patients and families work alongside healthcare providers to create a personalized plan that honors their values and preferences.

As we navigate the complexities of hospice care, it is essential to acknowledge the misconceptions that often surround it. Many people equate hospice with giving up or abandoning hope, viewing it as a last resort when all other treatment options have failed. This perception is rooted in a fear of death and a misunderstanding of the hospice philosophy. In reality, hospice is a proactive choice—a decision to prioritize comfort, dignity, and quality of life in the face of terminal illness. It is an affirmation of life, a recognition that even in the final stages, there are opportunities for joy, connection, and fulfillment. By reframing our understanding of hospice, we can begin to see it as a compassionate alternative to the often aggressive and invasive measures that characterize traditional medical care.

The role of hospice care extends beyond the individual and family; it also has implications for our broader society. As we grapple with an aging population and the increasing prevalence of chronic illnesses, the need for compassionate end-of-life care becomes ever more pressing. Hospice care challenges us to rethink our healthcare systems, advocating for a model that prioritizes patient-centered approaches and values the human experience. It calls for a shift in our cultural narrative around death, encouraging us to view it not as a taboo subject but as an integral part of the human experience. By fostering open discussions about death and dying, we can create a society that embraces the inevitability of mortality, allowing individuals to approach their final days with dignity and grace.

In conclusion, hospice care represents a compassionate alternative to the often harsh realities of modern medicine. It invites us to reimagine our relationship with death, encouraging us to embrace the beauty of life even in its final moments. By prioritizing comfort, dignity, and emotional support, hospice care empowers individuals to live fully until the end, creating a space where love, connection, and understanding can flourish. As we navigate the complexities of life and loss, let us remember the lessons of hospice: that every moment matters, that vulnerability can be a source of strength, and that the journey toward acceptance and peace is one we do not have to face alone. In the quiet embrace of hospice, we find not only a refuge from pain but also a celebration of life—a reminder that even in our final chapters, we can find meaning, connection, and love.

Chapter 18: Difficult Conversations: Breaking the Silence Around Death

In the quiet moments of our lives, when the world outside fades into a distant hum, we often confront the most profound truths of our existence. Death, that inevitable conclusion to our journey, remains a subject shrouded in silence, a topic few dare to broach openly. Yet, as we navigate the complexities of life, particularly in the face of terminal illness or the aging process, we find that these conversations, however difficult, are not just necessary; they can be transformative. The act of speaking about death can illuminate our fears, clarify our values, and ultimately lead us to a more peaceful acceptance of our mortality. It is a paradox that in confronting the end, we often discover a renewed appreciation for life itself.

The reluctance to discuss death is deeply ingrained in our culture. We are taught to avoid discomfort, to steer clear of topics that evoke fear or sadness. This aversion is understandable; death is not only the end of life but also the culmination of dreams, relationships, and aspirations. It represents a profound loss that can leave us feeling vulnerable and exposed. Yet, in our efforts to shield ourselves and our loved ones from pain, we may inadvertently prolong suffering. Conversations about death are not merely about the act of dying; they are about living fully and authentically. They provide an opportunity to reflect on what truly matters, to articulate our wishes, and to ensure that our voices are heard even when we can no longer speak for ourselves.

Initiating these conversations can feel daunting. The fear of upsetting loved ones, the worry of being misunderstood, or the anxiety of confronting our own mortality can create significant barriers. However, these discussions can also be a gift—an invitation to connect on a deeper level. When we approach the subject of death with honesty and compassion, we open the door to understanding and intimacy. It allows us to share our fears, our hopes, and our desires, creating a safe space for others to do the same. It is in this shared vulnerability that we can find strength and solidarity. As we gather around the table, sharing stories and memories, we can acknowledge the reality of our situation while also celebrating the richness of our lives.

One of the most challenging aspects of these conversations

is the emotional weight they carry. We may fear that discussing death will bring sadness or despair, but in truth, it can also foster a sense of clarity and purpose. When we articulate our values and wishes regarding end-of-life care, we empower ourselves and our loved ones to make informed decisions during times of crisis. This proactive approach can alleviate some of the burdens that accompany illness and dying. It allows us to define what a "good death" means to us, whether that involves remaining at home surrounded by loved ones, receiving palliative care, or exploring hospice options. By articulating these desires, we can ensure that our final days align with our values, allowing us to maintain a sense of agency even in the face of decline.

Moreover, these conversations can serve as a catalyst for healing. For many, the act of discussing death can unearth unresolved emotions, past grievances, and unspoken words. It provides an opportunity to mend relationships, express love, and seek forgiveness. As we confront the reality of our mortality, we are often reminded of the importance of connection and community. We may find ourselves reaching out to estranged family members, sharing our fears and hopes, and ultimately finding solace in the bonds we forge. These conversations can transform our relationships, allowing us to express gratitude, love, and understanding in ways that may have been previously unspoken.

In a healthcare context, the importance of having these

discussions cannot be overstated. Healthcare providers play a crucial role in facilitating conversations about death and dying, yet many hesitate to engage in these discussions, fearing they might take away hope. However, hope can take many forms. It can mean striving for a cure, but it can also mean finding peace, comfort, and dignity in the final stages of life. When healthcare professionals approach these conversations with empathy and openness, they can help patients and families navigate the complexities of end-of-life care. They can assist in clarifying treatment options, discussing goals of care, and ensuring that patients' wishes are honored.

As we consider the role of healthcare providers, it is essential to recognize that effective communication is a skill that can be cultivated. Training programs that focus on communication strategies can equip healthcare professionals with the tools they need to engage in difficult conversations. These programs can teach techniques for active listening, empathy, and compassion, enabling providers to create an environment where patients feel safe to express their fears and desires. By fostering a culture of open dialogue, we can break the silence surrounding death and encourage meaningful discussions that prioritize patient-centered care.

For families, initiating conversations about death can be just as vital. It is not uncommon for family members to avoid discussing end-of-life issues, fearing that such discussions may bring about an unwanted reality.

However, by engaging in these conversations, families can create a supportive atmosphere where everyone feels heard and valued. It is important to approach these discussions with sensitivity, acknowledging the emotions that may arise. Using open-ended questions can encourage dialogue, allowing family members to share their thoughts and feelings. Phrasing such as, "What are your thoughts about what you would want if you were unable to speak for yourself?" can open the door to deeper discussions about wishes and preferences.

In these conversations, it can be helpful to share personal experiences or stories of others who have navigated similar situations. By framing the discussion in a relatable context, we can help to normalize the conversation around death. It can also be beneficial to explore the values and beliefs that guide our perspectives on death. Discussing cultural or spiritual beliefs can provide a framework for understanding how different individuals approach the end of life, fostering empathy and respect for diverse viewpoints.

As we engage in these conversations, it is essential to remember that there is no right or wrong way to discuss death. Each individual and family will navigate this terrain differently, shaped by their unique experiences and beliefs. The key is to approach these discussions with an open heart and a willingness to listen. Allowing space for silence can also be powerful; sometimes, the most profound moments arise in the pauses between words. It is in these moments that we may find clarity, connection, and understanding.

Ultimately, the goal of these conversations is not to eliminate fear or sadness but to embrace the full spectrum of human experience. By acknowledging death as a natural part of life, we can cultivate a deeper appreciation for the time we have. We can learn to celebrate the small moments, to express love and gratitude, and to find joy in the connections we share. In confronting death, we often find a renewed sense of purpose and meaning, reminding us of the beauty that exists in our lives, even amid uncertainty.

As we reflect on the importance of breaking the silence around death, it becomes clear that these conversations are not merely about preparing for the end; they are about enriching our lives. They invite us to explore our values, to articulate our wishes, and to connect with our loved ones on a deeper level. They challenge us to confront our fears and embrace the vulnerability that comes with being human. In doing so, we can create a legacy of love, understanding, and acceptance that transcends the boundaries of life and death.

In the end, the most meaningful conversations about death are those that remind us of what it means to live fully. They encourage us to cherish our relationships, to express our feelings, and to embrace the present moment. By breaking the silence, we can transform our understanding of death from a source of fear into a catalyst for connection, healing, and ultimately, peace. So let us gather around the table, share our stories, and speak openly about the journey we all must face. In doing so, we honor not only our own lives but the lives of those we love, creating a tapestry of understanding that weaves through the fabric of our shared humanity.

Chapter 19 - The Legacy We Leave Behind: Creating Meaning in Final Days

As we navigate the often turbulent waters of life and death, the concept of legacy emerges as a vital beacon, guiding us toward a sense of purpose and fulfillment. Legacy is not merely about the tangible assets we leave behind; it encompasses the values we instill, the relationships we nurture, and the impact we have on the lives of others. In the final days of our lives, reflecting on our legacy can evoke a profound sense of clarity and urgency. It invites us to consider what truly matters and how we wish to be remembered. This contemplation can be a transformative experience, one that not only shapes our own understanding of meaning but also enriches the lives of those we hold dear.

Creating a meaningful legacy often begins with introspection. It requires us to look back at our lives, to sift through the myriad experiences that have shaped us. What moments stand out? What lessons have we learned? These reflections can illuminate the core values that define us—values such as love, kindness, integrity, and resilience. They serve as the foundation upon which we can build our legacy. In the face of mortality, these values can take on new significance. They remind us of the connections we have forged and the lives we have touched. For many, this process of reflection is not just about personal history; it is about the stories we share with others and the narratives that bind us together.

As we approach the end of life, the desire to communicate our legacy becomes increasingly urgent. We may find ourselves yearning to share our stories, to impart wisdom gleaned from a life well-lived. It is in these moments that the power of storytelling emerges as a vital tool for legacy creation. Sharing our narratives can foster intimacy and connection, allowing us to convey our values and beliefs to those we love. These stories become the threads that weave together the fabric of our relationships, creating a tapestry rich with meaning. Whether through conversation, letters, or recorded messages, the act of storytelling serves as a bridge between generations, ensuring that our essence endures long after we are gone.

In addition to storytelling, many individuals find solace in the act of creating tangible legacies. This can take various forms, from writing a memoir to establishing a charity or foundation that reflects our passions and values. These endeavors provide a concrete means of leaving a mark on the world, a way to ensure that our contributions continue to resonate. For example, a person passionate about education might choose to fund scholarships for underprivileged students, while another might dedicate their time to mentoring young people in their community. Such acts of generosity not only honor our values but also inspire others to carry forward the torch of our legacy. They create ripples of impact that extend far beyond our immediate circle, fostering a sense of continuity and connection.

Moreover, the legacy we leave behind is often intricately tied to the relationships we cultivate throughout our lives. In our final days, we may find ourselves reflecting on the people who have shaped our journey—those who have offered love, support, and companionship. These relationships are the true treasures of our existence, and nurturing them becomes paramount as we approach the end. It is essential to express gratitude, to acknowledge the ways in which others have enriched our lives. This can be a powerful act of closure, allowing us to leave behind not just memories but also a sense of love and appreciation that endures.

In the context of caregiving, the legacy we create can also extend to those who provide support during our final days. Caregivers often play a pivotal role in shaping our experiences, and acknowledging their contributions can be a meaningful way to honor our shared journey. Simple gestures of appreciation, such as heartfelt thank-you notes or shared moments of laughter, can leave an indelible mark on the hearts of those who care for us. By recognizing the humanity in our caregivers, we foster a sense of connection that transcends the caregiver-patient dynamic, creating a legacy of compassion and understanding.

As we contemplate our legacy, it is essential to recognize the role of forgiveness and reconciliation. In the shadow of death, unresolved conflicts and lingering grievances can weigh heavily on our hearts. The act of seeking forgiveness, whether from others or ourselves, can be a profound step toward healing. It allows us to release the burdens that may have held us captive for years, paving the way for a more peaceful farewell. In this context, legacy becomes not just about what we leave behind but also about the emotional and spiritual clarity we achieve in our final days. It invites us to let go of resentment and embrace love, creating a legacy that is rooted in compassion and understanding.

Furthermore, the legacy we create is often intertwined with the values we pass on to future generations. As we approach the end of life, we may find ourselves reflecting on the lessons we wish to impart to our children, grandchildren, and loved ones. It is an opportunity to share not only our successes but also our failures—the moments that shaped us and the insights we gained along the way. These conversations can be powerful catalysts for growth, encouraging younger generations to embrace their own journeys with courage and authenticity. By sharing our vulnerabilities, we empower others to navigate their own challenges with resilience, fostering a legacy of strength and wisdom.

In many cultures, rituals and ceremonies play a significant role in the process of legacy creation. These practices provide a structured way to honor our lives and the lives of those we love. Whether through memorial services, family gatherings, or personal rituals, these moments can serve as a powerful affirmation of our existence. They offer an opportunity for reflection, connection, and celebration, allowing us to acknowledge the impact we have had on others. In these gatherings, stories are shared, memories are cherished, and the threads of our legacy are woven together, creating a rich tapestry that honors the fullness of our lives.

As we explore the legacy we leave behind, it is crucial to embrace the concept of living fully until the end. The journey toward creating a meaningful legacy is not solely about the final days; it is about how we choose to live in the present. Each moment offers an opportunity to engage with the world, to connect with others, and to express our values. By cultivating a mindset of gratitude and presence, we can infuse our lives with purpose, ensuring that our legacy is not merely a reflection of our final days but a culmination of a life well-lived.

In this context, the act of embracing joy becomes a vital component of legacy creation. Even in the face of illness or impending death, moments of joy can be found in the simplest of experiences—a shared meal, a walk in nature, or a heartfelt conversation. These moments remind us of the beauty of life and the connections we hold dear. They serve as a testament to our resilience and our ability to find meaning in the midst of adversity. By prioritizing joy, we create a legacy that celebrates the richness of existence, encouraging others to seek out their own moments of happiness.

Ultimately, the legacy we leave behind is a reflection of the love we have shared, the values we have embodied, and the connections we have nurtured. It is a testament to the lives we have touched and the impact we have made on the world around us. As we approach our final days, we are given a unique opportunity to shape this legacy with intention and purpose. By embracing the power of storytelling, nurturing relationships, fostering forgiveness, and prioritizing joy, we can create a legacy that endures—a legacy that inspires others to live fully and authentically.

In the end, it is not the material possessions we accumulate or the accolades we achieve that define our legacy; it is the love we give, the kindness we extend, and the connections we forge. As we navigate the complexities of life and death, let us remember that our legacy is a living testament to the beauty of the human experience. It is an invitation to embrace our mortality with grace and to leave behind a legacy that resonates with meaning and purpose, reminding us all of the profound impact we can have on one another's lives.

Chapter 20: Planning Ahead: Legal and Practical Considerations for End-of-Life

In the quiet moments that precede a significant transition, a sense of urgency often emerges—an awareness that time is finite, that the choices we make today can reverberate through the lives of those we love. Planning ahead for end-of-life issues is not merely a practical necessity; it is an act of love, a way to ease the burdens of those we leave behind. It is about creating a roadmap that honors our values and wishes while also providing guidance for those who will navigate the terrain of grief and decision-making in our absence. The complexities of life, particularly as they pertain to death, can feel overwhelming, and yet, with a thoughtful approach, we can bring clarity to what might otherwise remain shrouded in uncertainty.

Legal considerations are often the first step in this journey of planning. Creating a will is a foundational act that ensures our assets are distributed according to our wishes. This document serves not only to delineate who receives what but also to affirm the relationships that have shaped our lives. It is an opportunity to express gratitude, to acknowledge those who have stood by us, and to leave behind a tangible reminder of our values. While the thought of discussing finances and possessions can feel uncomfortable, it is essential to confront these realities head-on. Engaging with a legal professional who specializes in estate planning can provide invaluable guidance, ensuring that our intentions are clearly articulated and legally binding. This process can also include the establishment of trusts, powers of attorney, and healthcare proxies, each serving a unique purpose in safeguarding our wishes and protecting our loved ones from unnecessary strife.

However, planning extends far beyond the realm of legal documents. It encompasses the more intimate aspects of our lives—the choices we make about our healthcare and the type of end-of-life care we desire. Conversations about these topics can be fraught with emotion, yet they are crucial in ensuring that our voices are heard, even when we can no longer speak for ourselves. Advance directives, which include living wills and durable powers of attorney for healthcare, allow us to articulate our preferences regarding medical treatment in the event that we become incapacitated. By documenting our wishes, we can prevent our loved ones from grappling with difficult decisions during an already painful time. It is a gift of clarity in moments of chaos, a way to alleviate the burden of choice from those who care for us.

The act of planning also invites us to reflect on the values that have guided our lives. What brings us joy? What defines a life well-lived? These questions can lead to profound insights, shaping the way we approach our final chapter. For some, this might mean prioritizing comfort and quality of life over aggressive medical interventions. For others, it may involve a desire to remain at home surrounded by loved ones, rather than in a sterile hospital environment. Engaging in these discussions with family members can foster a deeper understanding of one another's values and fears, creating a shared language around the often-taboo subject of death. It is an opportunity to connect, to share stories, and to reaffirm the bonds that unite us.

In many ways, planning ahead is an act of empowerment. It allows us to take control of our narrative, to dictate the terms of our departure rather than leaving it to chance. The fear of the unknown can be paralyzing, but by confronting it directly, we can find a sense of peace. This proactive approach not only benefits us but also provides reassurance to our loved ones. Knowing that we have made our wishes clear can alleviate some of the anxiety they may feel about making decisions on our behalf. It allows them to focus on what truly matters—being present, offering support, and cherishing the time we have together.

As we navigate the practicalities of end-of-life planning, it is essential to approach these conversations with sensitivity and compassion. Each family is unique, and the dynamics at play can significantly influence how discussions unfold. Some may find it easy to talk about death, while others may shy away from the topic altogether. It is vital to create a safe space for these conversations, where everyone feels heard and respected. This may involve multiple discussions over time, allowing individuals to process their feelings and come to terms with the realities of mortality at their own pace.

In addition to legal and healthcare considerations, we must also think about the emotional and spiritual dimensions of our end-of-life journey. What legacy do we want to leave behind? How do we wish to be remembered? These reflections can guide us in making choices that resonate with our core values. Creating a living legacy—whether through storytelling, art, or acts of service—can imbue our final days with purpose and meaning. It allows us to share our wisdom and experiences with those we love, offering them a tangible connection to our essence long after we are gone.

Moreover, planning ahead can also involve practical arrangements for our funeral or memorial service. While it may feel morbid to consider, having a clear plan can relieve our loved ones of the burden of making decisions during a time of grief. This might include specifying our preferences for burial or cremation, selecting readings or music that hold significance, or even outlining the tone we wish for the service. By taking these steps, we can ensure that our final farewell reflects our values and personality, creating a celebration of life rather than a somber occasion.

As we engage in the process of planning, it is crucial to revisit these discussions periodically. Life circumstances change, and our preferences may evolve as we journey through different stages. Regularly revisiting our advance directives, wills, and other legal documents ensures that they remain aligned with our current wishes. This practice not only affirms our commitment to living authentically but also reinforces the importance of open communication with our loved ones.

In the end, the act of planning ahead is a testament to our love and care for those we will leave behind. It is an acknowledgment of the fragility of life and the inevitability of death, wrapped in the hope that we can navigate this journey with grace and dignity. By addressing the practical, legal, emotional, and spiritual dimensions of end-of-life planning, we can create a framework that honors our values and provides comfort to those we cherish. In doing so, we not only prepare for our own passage but also gift our loved ones the assurance that they can carry our legacy forward with clarity and purpose. As we embrace the reality of mortality, we find the strength to live fully, to love deeply, and to leave behind a world enriched by our presence.

Chapter 21: Living Fully Until the End: Embracing Joy in Small Moments

In the final chapters of life, the notion of joy often feels like a distant echo, a fleeting thought that seems out of reach amid the shadows of uncertainty and fear. Yet, it is precisely in these moments of profound vulnerability that the potential for joy can be most transformative. The paradox of living fully until the end lies in our ability to embrace the small moments, to find beauty in the mundane, and to cultivate a sense of gratitude even when faced with the inevitable. This chapter invites you to explore the ways in which we can infuse our lives—and the lives of those we care for—with joy, no matter how limited our circumstances may seem.

Consider, for a moment, the simple act of sharing a meal.

For many, food is more than sustenance; it is an experience steeped in culture, memory, and connection. When a loved one is nearing the end of life, the ritual of eating together can take on a profound significance. It becomes a moment to pause, to reflect, and to celebrate the richness of life, even in its twilight. The flavors of a favorite dish, the laughter shared over a well-timed joke, or the warmth of a hand held across the table—these small moments can create a tapestry of joy that transcends the looming specter of mortality. It is in these gatherings that we can affirm life, acknowledge our shared humanity, and foster a sense of belonging that is often lost in the face of illness.

The power of presence cannot be underestimated. In a world that often feels rushed and disconnected, the act of simply being there for someone can be a profound source of comfort and joy. This presence does not require grand gestures or elaborate plans; it can be as simple as sitting quietly with a loved one, holding their hand, or engaging in a shared activity that brings them joy—whether it's listening to music, watching a favorite film, or reminiscing about cherished memories. These moments of connection remind us that joy is not solely found in the absence of pain or suffering, but in the deep, abiding relationships we cultivate throughout our lives. It is within these bonds that we can find solace and strength, even as we navigate the complexities of loss.

As caregivers, we often grapple with the weight of

responsibility, striving to provide the best care possible while managing our own emotional turmoil. Yet, amidst the demands of caregiving, it is crucial to carve out space for joy—not only for those we care for but for ourselves as well. This might mean allowing ourselves to indulge in small pleasures, whether it's enjoying a quiet moment with a cup of tea, taking a walk in nature, or engaging in a creative pursuit that brings us joy. By prioritizing our own well-being, we can better support our loved ones and create an environment that nurtures joy, even in the most challenging of circumstances.

In the face of terminal illness, it can be easy to succumb to a mindset of scarcity, where every moment feels overshadowed by grief and loss. However, embracing a mindset of abundance can help shift our perspective, allowing us to recognize the myriad of small joys that exist, even in the darkest of times. This might involve cultivating an attitude of gratitude, where we consciously acknowledge the beauty in the ordinary—the warmth of sunlight filtering through the window, the sound of laughter echoing in the hall, or the comfort of a soft blanket on a chilly evening. By training our minds to focus on these moments, we can create a reservoir of joy that sustains us and those around us.

Moreover, the act of sharing joy with others can be a powerful antidote to despair. When we engage in acts of kindness, whether big or small, we not only uplift others but also enrich our own lives. This could be as simple as writing a heartfelt note to a friend, surprising a loved one with their favorite dessert, or volunteering our time to support those in need. These gestures, while seemingly small, can create ripples of joy that extend far beyond our immediate circles, fostering a sense of community and connection that is vital in times of crisis.

As we navigate the complexities of end-of-life care, it is essential to remember that joy is not a denial of pain; rather, it coexists with it. It is entirely possible to experience joy and sorrow simultaneously, to laugh and to cry within the same breath. This duality is part of the human experience, and it is this complexity that makes life rich and meaningful. By allowing ourselves to feel both the weight of grief and the lightness of joy, we honor the full spectrum of our emotions and the depth of our experiences.

In many cultures, the concept of a "good death" is closely tied to the idea of living fully until the end. This notion encompasses the idea that, regardless of our circumstances, we have the power to shape our final days in ways that reflect our values, our passions, and our relationships. This might involve creating a legacy of joy, where we actively seek to share happiness with those we love, imparting lessons of resilience and gratitude that will endure long after we are gone. By prioritizing joy in our final moments, we can leave behind a narrative that celebrates life rather than one that is solely focused on loss.

As we reflect on the journey of living fully until the end, it is essential to recognize that joy is not a destination; it is a practice—a conscious choice to seek out the beauty in our lives, no matter how fleeting. It is about learning to be present, to savor each moment, and to find meaning in the simple pleasures that surround us. This practice can be cultivated through mindfulness, where we train ourselves to observe our thoughts and feelings without judgment, allowing us to fully engage with the present moment and appreciate the richness of our experiences.

In the context of caregiving, this practice of mindfulness can be particularly powerful. It invites us to slow down, to breathe, and to fully immerse ourselves in the experience of caring for another. By approaching caregiving with a sense of presence and intention, we can create an atmosphere of joy that permeates our interactions, transforming even the most mundane tasks into opportunities for connection and love. Whether it's preparing a meal, administering medication, or simply sitting in silence, these moments can become sacred when approached with mindfulness and gratitude.

Ultimately, the journey of living fully until the end is one of embracing the complexity of life—of acknowledging that joy and sorrow can coexist, that love can flourish even in the face of loss, and that every moment is an opportunity to create meaning. As we navigate the challenges of caregiving and end-of-life decisions, let us remember that joy is not something to be sought after; it is something to be cultivated, nurtured, and shared. It is in the small moments—the laughter shared, the stories told, the love expressed—that we can find a sense of peace and fulfillment, even as we face the unknown.

In the end, let us strive to live fully, to embrace joy in its many forms, and to honor the lives we touch with our presence and love. As we journey through the complexities of life, loss, and the quest for peace, may we find solace in the knowledge that joy is always within reach, waiting to be discovered in the most unexpected of places.

Chapter 22 - The Gift of Letting Go: Finding Freedom in Acceptance

In the journey of life, there comes a moment when we are confronted with the profound reality of letting go. This is not merely about relinquishing physical possessions or even the relationships that have shaped us; it is about embracing the inherent impermanence of existence itself. Letting go can be one of the most difficult tasks we face, especially when it involves those we love or the dreams we have nurtured for years. Yet, in the act of letting go, we often discover a remarkable freedom—an opportunity to redefine our relationship with loss, to transform our grief into a deeper understanding of what it means to live fully. Acceptance is not a destination; it is a process, a gradual unfolding that requires patience, courage, and an openness to the lessons that life, in its unpredictable nature, has to offer.

As we navigate the complexities of life and death, we may find ourselves clinging to the past, to memories that have shaped our identity and our sense of belonging. This clinging is a natural response to fear—the fear of losing what we hold dear, the fear of the unknown that lies ahead. However, the paradox of attachment is that it can lead to suffering. When we resist the inevitable changes that life presents, we often find ourselves trapped in a cycle of pain and longing. The process of letting go invites us to confront this fear head-on, to acknowledge the reality of our circumstances without judgment. It encourages us to recognize that while we cannot control the events of our lives, we can choose how we respond to them. In this choice lies the key to our liberation.

Letting go does not mean forgetting; rather, it involves a shift in perspective. It is about honoring the memories and experiences that have enriched our lives while allowing ourselves the grace to move forward. This can be particularly poignant in the context of caregiving and end-of-life decisions. As caregivers, we often find ourselves in a position where we must confront our loved ones' mortality. The weight of this responsibility can feel overwhelming, yet it is in this very challenge that we can discover profound opportunities for connection, empathy, and understanding. By embracing the reality of our loved one's declining health, we create space for meaningful conversations about their wishes, their fears, and their hopes for the time they have left. In these moments, we learn that letting go can also mean relinquishing the need to control the outcome, to fix what cannot be mended.

In the face of terminal illness, we are often thrust into a whirlwind of emotions—fear, sadness, anger, and even moments of joy. Each of these feelings is valid, and each offers us a unique lens through which to view our situation. When we allow ourselves to feel deeply, we open the door to acceptance. This acceptance is not an act of resignation; rather, it is a conscious choice to acknowledge the reality of our circumstances while still finding ways to celebrate life. It is through this lens that we can begin to appreciate the beauty of small moments—the laughter shared over a favorite memory, the quiet companionship of sitting together in silence, the warmth of a hand held in solidarity. These moments become the fabric of our shared experience, a testament to the love that endures even in the face of loss.

The act of letting go also invites us to reflect on our own lives. It challenges us to consider what we truly value and what we wish to carry forward. Often, we find ourselves burdened by the weight of expectations—our own or those imposed by society. In the context of caregiving, this can manifest as a relentless drive to "do it all," to ensure that our loved ones have every possible comfort and care. Yet, in the pursuit of this ideal, we may overlook the importance of our own well-being. Letting go of the notion that we must be perfect caregivers allows us to embrace our humanity. It reminds us that we, too, are deserving of compassion, rest, and support. In acknowledging our limitations, we create room for authenticity in our relationships, fostering a deeper connection with those we care for.

As we journey through the process of acceptance, we may encounter the resistance of those around us. Friends and family may struggle to let go, clinging to hope or denial as a means of coping with the impending loss. In these moments, it is essential to approach the situation with empathy and understanding. Each person's journey toward acceptance is unique, shaped by their experiences, beliefs, and coping mechanisms. By offering a compassionate presence, we can create an environment that encourages open dialogue about the realities of our situation. It is through these conversations that we can collectively navigate the complexities of grief, allowing ourselves to grieve not only for what is being lost but also for what has been shared.

In the context of hospice care, the philosophy of letting go takes on an even deeper significance. Hospice embodies the belief that every moment matters, that life should be lived fully until the very end. This perspective encourages patients and their families to shift their focus from the fight against illness to the celebration of life. It invites us to let go of the fear of death and to embrace the beauty of living in the present. In hospice settings, patients are often encouraged to reflect on their lives, to share their stories, and to engage in meaningful activities that bring them joy. This process of reflection can be transformative, allowing individuals to find peace in their choices and to let go of regrets that may have lingered for years.

The gift of letting go ultimately lies in the freedom it offers. When we release our grip on what we cannot change, we create space for new possibilities. We begin to see that acceptance does not diminish our love or our memories; rather, it enhances them. In letting go, we honor the journey we have shared with our loved ones, recognizing that their essence will forever remain a part of us. This understanding can be a source of comfort as we navigate the complexities of grief. It allows us to carry forward the lessons learned, the love shared, and the moments cherished, even as we mourn the physical absence of those we hold dear.

As we approach the conclusion of our journey together, let us remember that the act of letting go is not a sign of weakness; it is an affirmation of our resilience. It is a testament to our ability to adapt, to grow, and to find meaning in the face of adversity. In embracing the gift of letting go, we open ourselves to the beauty of life in all its forms. We learn to appreciate the fleeting moments, to find joy in the mundane, and to cultivate gratitude for the experiences that have shaped us. This journey toward acceptance is a deeply personal one, yet it is also a universal experience that connects us all. In sharing our stories, in leaning on one another, we find solace in the knowledge that we are not alone.

In the end, letting go becomes a celebration of life—a recognition that while our loved ones may no longer be physically present, their impact endures in the hearts and minds of those they touched. It is a reminder that love transcends the boundaries of time and space, that the bonds we create are unbreakable, even in the face of loss. As we learn to navigate the complexities of grief, may we find the courage to let go, to embrace acceptance, and to live fully in every moment that remains. In doing so, we honor not only ourselves but also the legacies of those we hold dear, weaving their memories into the tapestry of our lives as we continue to journey forward.

Chapter 23 - Guiding Loved Ones Through Grief and Bereavement

When we think of grief, we often envision a solitary journey, a path walked in silence, marked by the absence of the one we have lost. Yet, the reality is that grief is a communal experience, one that intertwines the lives of those left behind. This chapter seeks to illuminate how we can guide our loved ones through their grief, offering support and companionship in a time that can feel profoundly isolating. Grief is not merely an emotional response; it is a process that encompasses a wide range of feelings, from sorrow and anger to confusion and even relief. Understanding this complexity is crucial for anyone who finds themselves in the role of a supporter. It is essential to recognize that each person's grief is unique, shaped by their relationship with the deceased, their personal history, and their coping mechanisms. Therefore, our approach must be flexible, empathetic, and attuned to the individual needs of those we are trying to help.

At the heart of guiding others through grief is the act of listening—truly listening. In a society that often rushes to fill silence with platitudes or well-meaning but superficial reassurances, we must resist the urge to minimize another's pain. Instead, we should create a space where feelings can be expressed freely. This means allowing the bereaved to share their memories, their regrets, and their hopes without fear of judgment or dismissal. Sometimes, the most powerful thing we can do is to simply be present, offering our silent companionship as they navigate the tumultuous waters of their emotions. We should remind ourselves that grief is not a linear process; it does not follow a predictable timeline, and it cannot be hurried. Each wave of grief may bring with it a new set of emotions that can feel overwhelming. Our role is not to fix this but to sit with them in their discomfort, to acknowledge their pain, and to validate their experience.

In addition to being present, we can also help by encouraging our loved ones to share their feelings with others. Grief can often feel like a burdensome secret, one that the bereaved feel they must carry alone. By gently suggesting they reach out to friends, family, or support groups, we can help them understand that they are not alone in their sorrow. Sharing stories about the deceased can be a healing process, allowing the bereaved to keep the memory alive while also processing their loss. It is vital to create an environment where these conversations can happen naturally, perhaps by inviting others to share their own memories or by reminiscing together about shared experiences. This act of storytelling can transform grief into a celebration of life, allowing those left behind to find comfort in the shared love they all had for the deceased.

As we guide our loved ones through grief, we must also be mindful of the physical aspects of support. Grief can manifest in physical ways—fatigue, loss of appetite, and even physical pain. Offering practical help can be just as important as emotional support. This might mean preparing meals, assisting with household chores, or simply being there to help with day-to-day tasks that may feel overwhelming. The act of caregiving in this way can alleviate some of the burdens that come with grief, allowing the bereaved to focus on their emotional healing. It is also important to check in regularly, reminding them that we are there for them, even if they may not feel like talking. A simple text message or phone call can serve as a lifeline, a reminder that they are not forgotten and that their grief is acknowledged.

However, as we extend our support, we must also be aware of the boundaries of our role. It is easy to want to take on the weight of another's grief, to feel responsible for their healing. Yet, we must remember that grief is ultimately a personal journey, one that each person must navigate in their own way. It is essential to encourage our loved ones to seek professional help if their grief becomes too overwhelming or if they show signs of complicated grief, such as prolonged despair or an inability to function in daily life. Suggesting therapy or counseling can provide them with additional tools to cope, reinforcing the idea that seeking help is not a sign of weakness but a step toward healing.

In the wake of loss, the world can feel stark and unforgiving. The rituals surrounding death—funerals, memorial services, and even the quiet moments of remembrance—can serve as crucial touchpoints in the grieving process. These rituals provide a framework for expressing sorrow and honoring the deceased. Encouraging participation in these rituals can help the bereaved find a sense of closure, even if that closure is imperfect. It is important to remember that grief does not have a set endpoint; it evolves over time, often resurfacing in unexpected ways. By acknowledging this reality, we can help our loved ones understand that it is okay to feel joy while also feeling sadness, that they can carry the memory of their loved one with them while still moving forward in their own lives.

One of the most profound aspects of grief is the way it can transform relationships. As we support those who are grieving, we may find our own feelings of loss surfacing, as we remember our connections with the deceased. This shared experience of grief can deepen bonds, creating a sense of solidarity among those left behind. It can also serve as a reminder of our own mortality, prompting us to reflect on our relationships and the legacies we wish to leave behind. In this way, grief can act as a catalyst for growth, encouraging us to cherish our connections and to express our love more openly.

As we navigate the complexities of guiding loved ones through grief, we must also be mindful of our own emotional well-being. Supporting someone in their grief can be emotionally taxing, and it is crucial to practice self-care. By ensuring that we are taking care of our own needs, we can be more effective in our support of others. This might mean seeking our own sources of solace, whether through friends, hobbies, or even professional support. When we are grounded in our own emotional health, we are better equipped to offer the compassion and understanding that those who are grieving so desperately need.

Ultimately, guiding loved ones through grief is an act of love, one that requires patience, empathy, and an open heart. It is a journey that invites us to confront our own feelings about loss and mortality, while also providing us with the opportunity to forge deeper connections with those we care about. In a world that often shies away from discussions about death, we can become beacons of support, helping to normalize the conversation around grief and loss. By doing so, we honor not only the memories of those we have lost but also the resilience of the human spirit, which can find a way to heal, even in the face of profound sorrow. As we walk alongside our loved ones in their darkest moments, we can help illuminate a path toward healing, reminding them that while grief may be a part of their journey, it does not have to define it.

Chapter 24 - A Better Ending: Designing a Death That Aligns with Your Values

In our society, death is often a topic shrouded in discomfort and avoidance, a subject we tend to sidestep in conversation, as if the mere mention of it could invite misfortune. Yet, death is as intrinsic to the human experience as birth, and understanding it can be a profound journey toward living fully. When we confront the reality of our mortality, we are given a unique opportunity to reflect on our values, to distill our lives into what truly matters. This process is not merely about preparing for an end; it is about enriching the entirety of our existence. Designing a death that aligns with our values requires us to engage in honest dialogues with ourselves and those we love, to articulate what we cherish most, and to ensure that our final moments resonate with the essence of who we are.

The conversation surrounding end-of-life choices often begins with a stark realization: we are not invincible. A diagnosis, an accident, or even the natural progression of aging can thrust us into a space where we must make decisions that will shape the latter chapters of our lives. Yet, grappling with these realities can be daunting. Many of us may feel overwhelmed by the medical jargon, the myriad options for treatment, or the emotional weight of the decisions we face. It is in these moments that we must reclaim agency over our lives and deaths. We must ask ourselves what kind of experience we want in our final days. Do we wish to be surrounded by family in a familiar setting, or would we prefer the sterile comfort of a hospital room? What are our beliefs about suffering, and how do they inform our choices? By answering these questions, we begin to craft an ending that is not only bearable but deeply meaningful.

To design a death that reflects our values, we must first articulate those values. This process often requires introspection and vulnerability. What brings us joy? What gives our lives meaning? For some, it may be the simple pleasures of a shared meal with loved ones, the laughter of grandchildren, or the quiet moments spent in nature. For others, it may be the pursuit of knowledge, creativity, or spiritual fulfillment. By identifying these core values, we can begin to envision how we want to experience the end of our lives. Perhaps we wish to prioritize comfort over aggressive treatment, or maybe we seek to leave a legacy through our stories and wisdom. Whatever our values may be, they serve as a compass, guiding us through the complex landscape of end-of-life choices.

Conversations about death and dying can be uncomfortable, yet they are essential to ensuring our wishes are honored. Initiating these discussions with family members can be challenging, but it is a critical step in the process. Sharing our desires and fears can deepen our connections, allowing our loved ones to understand our perspectives and support us in our choices. It is important to recognize that these conversations do not have to be morbid; they can be infused with love, humor, and a sense of purpose. We can frame our discussions around the legacy we wish to leave, the memories we cherish, and the values we hold dear. By doing so, we create an environment where everyone feels safe to express their thoughts and emotions, fostering a sense of unity as we navigate this inevitable journey together.

As we engage in these conversations, we may also encounter differing opinions and beliefs about death and dying. Family members may have their own ideas about what constitutes a "good" death, shaped by their experiences and cultural backgrounds. It is essential to approach these differences with empathy and openness. Listening to one another's perspectives can illuminate the diverse ways in which we process the concept of mortality. We may find that our loved ones have insights that resonate with us, or we may discover that our values are not as aligned as we believed. In either case, the act of sharing and listening can enrich our understanding of what it means to live and die well.

Another critical aspect of designing a death that aligns with our values is understanding the medical landscape in which we find ourselves. The healthcare system can be bewildering, filled with jargon, protocols, and a plethora of choices that can leave us feeling disoriented. It is crucial to educate ourselves about our options, whether that involves palliative care, hospice services, or advanced directives. Each of these avenues offers different approaches to end-of-life care, and understanding them can empower us to make informed decisions. Palliative care focuses on alleviating suffering and improving quality of life, regardless of the stage of illness, while hospice care provides specialized support for those nearing the end of life. Advanced directives, such as living wills and healthcare proxies, allow us to articulate our wishes regarding medical treatment and appoint someone to make decisions on our behalf if we are unable to do so. By familiarizing ourselves with these concepts, we can approach our healthcare providers with confidence, ensuring that our values are respected in our care.

In the midst of these discussions and decisions, it is essential to cultivate a sense of peace and acceptance. The journey toward the end of life can be fraught with anxiety and uncertainty, but finding ways to embrace the present moment can provide solace. Mindfulness practices, such as meditation or gentle yoga, can help us center ourselves and cultivate a deeper awareness of our thoughts and feelings. Engaging in creative pursuits, such as writing, painting, or music, can also offer an outlet for expression and reflection. These practices can serve as reminders that even in the face of mortality, there is beauty and meaning to be found in the here and now.

As we navigate the complexities of end-of-life choices, it is vital to remember that we are not alone. Many resources are available to support us in this journey, from hospice organizations to community groups focused on death and dying. Engaging with these resources can provide valuable information, emotional support, and a sense of connection with others who share similar experiences. Additionally, seeking the guidance of professionals, such as social workers or chaplains, can offer a compassionate ear and help us process our emotions as we confront the realities of mortality.

Ultimately, designing a death that aligns with our values is an act of love—both for ourselves and for those we leave behind. It is an opportunity to reflect on our lives, to share our stories, and to impart our wisdom. By engaging in this process, we can create a legacy that transcends our physical existence, allowing our loved ones to carry forward the essence of who we are. In this way, death becomes not an end but a continuation—a thread woven into the fabric of life that connects us to those we cherish.

As we embark on this journey, let us remember that the choices we make today can shape the experience of our final days. By embracing the reality of our mortality, we can live more fully, savoring each moment and nurturing our connections with others. Let us approach the end of life not with fear, but with an open heart, ready to embrace the beauty of our shared humanity. In doing so, we can transform our understanding of death from a source of dread into a poignant reminder of the richness of life itself. Through this lens, we can design a death that honors our values, reflects our true selves, and ultimately allows us to find peace in the journey we all must undertake.

Chapter 25 - The Journey Beyond Loss: Hope and Renewal After Goodbye

In the quiet aftermath of loss, when the world feels like it has dimmed and the familiar rhythms of life have been disrupted, we often find ourselves grappling with a profound sense of emptiness. The death of a loved one, whether sudden or anticipated, leaves an indelible mark on our lives, reshaping our understanding of what it means to exist and to love. As we navigate this tumultuous terrain, we are confronted with a series of questions that can feel overwhelming: How do we carry on in the absence of those we hold dear? What does it mean to find hope in the wake of grief? And perhaps most importantly, how can we honor the memories of those we have lost while also allowing ourselves to heal and grow? These questions do not have easy answers, but they are essential to the journey of finding meaning and renewal after goodbye.

Grief is a complex and deeply personal experience, often characterized by a myriad of emotions that can shift from one moment to the next. We may find ourselves feeling anger, sadness, guilt, and even relief, all swirling together in a confusing mix that can leave us feeling isolated. Each person's journey through grief is unique, shaped by the nature of the relationship we had with the deceased, the circumstances surrounding their death, and our own coping mechanisms. In this way, grief is not a linear process, but rather a winding path that can take us to unexpected places. It is essential to remind ourselves that there is no right or wrong way to grieve; there is only our way. Embracing this truth can be liberating, allowing us to honor our feelings without judgment and to give ourselves permission to experience the full range of emotions that accompany loss.

As we navigate our grief, we may also find ourselves reflecting on the lives of those we have lost—their joys, their struggles, their dreams. In these moments of remembrance, we can find a sense of connection that transcends death. It is in our stories and shared experiences that we keep our loved ones alive within us. We may choose to create rituals or memorials that celebrate their lives, whether that means lighting a candle, sharing stories with friends and family, or even engaging in activities that they loved. These acts of remembrance can serve as powerful reminders of the love that continues to exist, even in the absence of physical presence. They can help us to forge a new relationship with our grief, one that acknowledges the pain but also honors the beauty of what was shared.

While the journey of grief can feel isolating, it is important to remember that we are not alone. Many people walk this path, and there are communities and resources available to support us. Whether through support groups, therapy, or simply leaning on friends and family, seeking connection can be a vital part of healing. Sharing our experiences with others who understand can provide solace and validation, reminding us that our feelings are not only normal but also shared by many. In these spaces, we can find the strength to express our grief, to cry, to laugh, and to remember. We can also learn from others who have navigated similar journeys, gaining insights into how they found hope and renewal after their own losses.

Hope, in the context of grief, is often misunderstood. It does not mean the absence of pain or the quick return to normalcy; rather, it is the quiet resilience that allows us to envision a future where joy can coexist with sorrow. Hope can manifest in small, everyday moments—a smile from a stranger, a sunset that takes our breath away, or a memory that brings both laughter and tears. It is the gentle reminder that life continues, and with it, the possibility for new experiences and connections. Cultivating hope requires us to be patient with ourselves, to recognize that healing is not a destination but a journey. It is about finding ways to integrate our loss into our lives, allowing it to shape us without defining us.

As we begin to find our footing in this new reality, we may also discover a renewed sense of purpose. Loss can be a catalyst for change, prompting us to reevaluate our values, our relationships, and our aspirations. In the wake of grief, we may feel compelled to honor the legacy of our loved ones by living more fully ourselves. This could mean pursuing a long-held dream, advocating for a cause they were passionate about, or simply making a conscious effort to savor the small moments of joy in our daily lives. By embracing the lessons learned from our losses, we can create a life that reflects both our own desires and the memory of those we cherish.

The journey beyond loss is also an opportunity for introspection and growth. It invites us to examine our own beliefs about life, death, and everything in between. We may find ourselves pondering the meaning of existence and the impact we wish to leave on the world. This existential questioning can be uncomfortable, but it can also lead to profound insights about what truly matters to us. Engaging with these questions can help us to clarify our values and priorities, guiding us toward a more intentional way of living. As we confront our mortality, we are reminded of the preciousness of time and the importance of making choices that align with our authentic selves.

In this journey, we must also acknowledge the role of

self-compassion. Grief can be accompanied by feelings of guilt or regret, particularly if we believe we could have done more for our loved ones or if we struggle to find joy in the wake of their passing. It is crucial to approach ourselves with kindness during this time, recognizing that we are doing the best we can in an incredibly difficult situation. Self-compassion allows us to sit with our pain without judgment, to give ourselves grace as we navigate the complexities of grief. It is a reminder that we are worthy of love and care, even in our darkest moments.

As we move forward, we may also find solace in the natural world. Nature has a remarkable ability to heal and restore, offering us a sense of peace and perspective that can be difficult to find elsewhere. Whether it is through a walk in the park, tending to a garden, or simply sitting quietly in a natural setting, immersing ourselves in the beauty of the world around us can provide a much-needed respite from our grief. The cycles of nature—birth, growth, decay, and renewal—mirror our own experiences and remind us that life continues, even in the face of loss. In these moments, we can find a sense of connection to something greater than ourselves, a reminder that we are part of a vast and intricate tapestry of life.

Ultimately, the journey beyond loss is not about forgetting or moving on; it is about finding a way to carry our loved ones with us as we navigate the complexities of our own lives. It is about learning to live in a world that feels different, yet still holds the potential for beauty and joy. As we honor the memories of those we have lost, we can also embrace the possibilities that lie ahead. In this delicate balance of remembrance and renewal, we can begin to forge a new path—one that acknowledges our grief while also celebrating the resilience of the human spirit.

In the end, the journey beyond loss is a testament to the power of love. It is a reminder that while death may separate us physically, the bonds we share with those we cherish can never be broken. As we navigate this journey, let us hold onto the lessons learned, the memories cherished, and the hope that sustains us. In doing so, we can create a life that honors our loved ones and reflects the fullness of our own humanity—a life that embraces both the light and the shadows, the joy and the sorrow, as we continue to seek meaning in every chapter of our existence.

Manufactured by Amazon.ca
Acheson, AB